Praise from Reviewers...

"Dr. William Manger and Dr. Ray Gifford, two of the most experienced and distinguished clinician-scientists and hypertension specialists in the nation, have come to the rescue. Their book *100 Questions and Answers about Hypertension* provides easy access to the information we need to better understand and deal with high blood pressure. It should be required reading for anyone who has high blood pressure or cares for those who have it.

We have developed methods to diagnose and treat hypertension, and we have proven that treatment saves lives. Now we have to get this news to all. Manger and Gifford have made this task much easier."

— *Henry R. Black, MD*
Charles J. and Margaret Robert Professor
Chairman, Preventive Medicine
Professor, Internal Medicine
Rush-Presbyterian-St. Luke's Medical Center
Chicago, Illinois

"This book, written by two experts in the field of hypertension with almost 100 years of experience between them, is a storehouse of information that will be useful to all who have (or live with people who have) high blood pressure. The chapters are brief, easily understood and thorough in covering every important feature of this condition. The advice is practical and attainable, reflecting the authors' immense clinical experience."

— *Norman M. Kaplan, MD*
Professor of Medicine
University of Texas

"Doctors William Manger and Ray Gifford Jr. are well-known and experienced clinicians in the field of hypertension. After many years of their independent medical practice they have been confronted by a multitude of questions by their patients. This volume organizes these questions of the concerned reader and provides, in easy to understand answers, their considered responses in a non-controversial and straightforward manner."

— *Edward D. Frohlich, MD*
Alton Ochsner Distinguished Scientist
Alton Ochsner Medical Foundation
Editor-in-Chief, Hypertension

"100 pearls about high blood pressure for the lay person and physician alike."

— *Francis Haddy, MD, PhD*
Past President American Physiological Society
and NASA Life Sciences Advisory Committee
and Professor and Chairman Emeritus
Department of Physiology
USUHS Medical School

"The book *100 Questions and Answers about Hypertension* by Drs. William Manger and Ray Gifford Jr. is an extraordinary find to any hypertension patient and their family. It is like having a 2–3 hour consultation with your internist; a nice idea, but unlikely to happen. This book makes it happen. It covers every possible question on hypertension and more. Most non-hypertension physicians could not begin to detail the various hypertension drugs, their benefits, and side effects that Drs. Manger and Gifford have catalogued in their book. In addition, the style and language are easily understandable by those without any medical background. It is truly a bible for all hypertension patients."

— *Richard J. Coburn, DMD, MD*
  Attending, Beth Israel Hospital, New York City

"Drs. Manger and Gifford have done a superb job in addressing the most important issues in the field of hypertension for the layperson. Written in a question-and-answer format, the text provides information in a way that is thoughtful, erudite, understandable, and educational. I recommend this text for any layperson, or for physicians to share with their patients who seek a better understanding of the problem of hypertension. It is a very useful and well-written work that should serve the public well."

— *Joseph Loscalzo, MD, PhD*
  Wade Professor and Chairman
  Department of Medicine
  Director, Whitaker Cardiovascular Institute
  Boston University School of Medicine
  Boston, Massachusetts

"Timely and authoritative advice from two of the leading experts in the field."

— *Thomas Pickering, MD*
  Professor of Medicine
  Hypertension Center
  New York Hospital—Cornell Medical Center

"The need for effective educational methods in health science is greater today than ever before given the amount of new information available. I fully endorse the authors' efforts to provide a new vehicle to 'get the message out' that blood pressure control is of paramount importance. Drs. Manger and Gifford are two of the most experienced and respected clinician scientists in our field and their perspectives are extremely valuable."

— *Joseph L. Izzo, Jr., MD*
  Professor of Medicine, SUNY—Buffalo
  Co-Editor, Hypertension Primer

For Stuart and Michelle Feinstein
with very best wishes
Bill Manger
1/20/04

100 Questions and Answers about Hypertension

100 Questions and Answers about Hypertension

By

William M. Manger, MD, PhD
Professor of Clinical Medicine
New York University Medical Center
Chairman, National Hypertension Association
New York, New York

Ray W. Gifford, Jr., MD
Emeritus Chairman
Department of Hypertension/Nephrology
Cleveland Clinic
Cleveland, Ohio
President, National Hypertension Association
New York, New York

Blackwell
Science

© 2001 by Blackwell Science, Inc.

Editorial Offices:
Commerce Place, 350 Main Street, Malden, Massachusetts 02148, USA
Osney Mead, Oxford OX2 0EL, England
25 John Street, London WC1N 2BL, England
23 Ainslie Place, Edinburgh EH3 6AJ, Scotland
54 University Street, Carlton, Victoria 3053, Australia

Other Editorial Offices:
Blackwell Wissenschafts-Verlag GmbH, Kurfürstendamm 57, 10707 Berlin, Germany
Blackwell Science KK, MG Kodenmacho Building, 7-10 Kodenmacho Nihombashi, Chuo-ku, Tokyo 104, Japan

Distributors:

USA
Blackwell Science, Inc.
Commerce Place
350 Main Street
Malden, Massachusetts 02148
(Telephone orders: 800-215-1000
or 781-388-8250;
fax orders: 781-388-8270)

Canada
Login Brothers Book Company
324 Saulteaux Crescent
Winnipeg, Manitoba R3J 3T2
(Telephone orders: 204-837-2987)

Australia
Blackwell Science Pty, Ltd.
54 University Street
Carlton, Victoria 3053
(Telephone orders: 03-9347-0300;
fax orders: 03-9349-3016)

Outside North America and Australia
Blackwell Science, Ltd.
c/o Marston Book Services, Ltd.
P.O. Box 269
Abingdon
Oxon OX14 4YN
England
(Telephone orders: 44-01235-465500;
fax orders: 44-01235-465555)

All rights reserved. No part of this book may be reproduced in any form or by any electronic or mechanical means, including information storage and retrieval systems, without permission in writing from the publisher, except by a reviewer who may quote brief passages in a review.

Acquisitions: Chris Davis
Development: Julia Casson
Production: Erin Whitehead
Manufacturing: Lisa Flanagan
Marketing Manager: Anne Stone
Cover design by Leslie Haimes
Interior design by Eve Siegel

Typeset by Best-set Typesetter Ltd., Hong Kong
Printed and bound by Capital City Press

Printed in the United States of America
02 03 5 4 3

The Blackwell Science logo is a trade mark of Blackwell Science Ltd., registered at the United Kingdom Trade Marks Registry.

Library of Congress Cataloging-in-Publication Data

Manger, William Muir, 1920–
    100 questions and answers about hypertension / by William M. Manger and Ray W. Gifford.
        p.   cm.
    ISBN 0-632-04481-0
    1. Hypertension—Miscellanea.   2. Hypertension—Popular works.   I. Title: One hundred questions and answers about hypertension.   II. Gifford, Ray W. (Ray Wallace), 1923–III. Title.

RC685.H8   M277 2001
616.1'32—dc21   00-056422

To our mentors in hypertension
at the Mayo and Cleveland Clinics:
Edgar van Nuys Allen, MD
Irvine Heinly Page, MD

"We can see farther than the ancients not because we have better vision or greater stature, but because we have been lifted up by giants."
—Bernard De Chartres
12th century philosopher

Contents

Foreword

Drs. Ray W. Gifford, Jr. and William Manger are answering the call to help us address a very important public health problem—i.e., waning public knowledge and control of high blood pressure. Their informative book comes none too soon because the national effort to control hypertension, the medical term for high blood pressure, appears to be ebbing. Despite progress over the last 30 years, hypertension control rates are no longer improving, and we have not reached the Department of Health and Human Services millennium goal to bring 50% of Americans afflicted with hypertension under control. Subsequently the reductions in heart disease and stroke are not as large as we have become accustomed to seeing. Today, hypertension is the primary factor in the deaths of more than 2,000,000 Americans each year. Hypertension precedes heart failure in 90% of all cases and the prevalence of heart failure, greater today than ten years ago, is now the largest single component of the Medicare budget. Cardiovascular diseases cost the nation more than 316 billion dollars each year. Unlike so many other medical conditions for which we have limited treatment options, hypertension, the leading cause of heart disease and stroke, is easily detectable and usually controllable. This book, which contains clear and concise information, is a valuable tool for patients to use with their doctor since both work to prevent and control this condition. Today's treatments for controlling hypertension are many and excellent. When applied, they produce remarkable results. Studies have shown that controlling hypertension can reduce strokes by 40%, heart attacks by 25%, and heart failure by more than 50%. And because 50 million Americans have high blood pressure, it is clear that controlling this condition has profound consequences. So once again, we are indebted to Drs. Gifford and Manger, two outstanding scientists, physicians, and teachers, for taking the time to help the public understand some very important health issues. With this book you, and your doctor, have what it takes to prevent and control high blood pressure.

Edward J. Roccella, PhD, MPH
Coordinator
National High Blood Pressure Education Program

Preface

The magnitude of the hypertension (high blood pressure) problem in the United States and most of the world is enormous! An estimated 50 million Americans have hypertension—nearly one of every four adults—and hypertension is the most common reason for seeing a physician. This condition is a major contributor to both heart disease and stroke. Approximately 1.1 million Americans suffer heart attacks annually, and nearly one-third of those victims die; 600,000 strokes occur annually, of which 160,000 prove fatal.

Hypertension is a major contributor to cardiovascular disease (stroke, heart attack, heart and kidney failure, and hardening of the arteries), which is the leading cause of death in the United States. Cardiovascular disease kills almost 1 million people each year, and it cripples and disables the same number of people. In addition, it is the most important source of invalidism and lost workdays because of brain, heart, and kidney damage, being responsible for more than 52 million workdays of lost productivity. One-half of all hypertensives are members of the work force, and 34% of the work force has high blood pressure or borderline elevations of blood pressure.

Approximately 75% of all stroke victims have high blood pressure, and strokes cost Americans $45 billion in medical bills and lost earnings each year. The average lifetime cost of a stroke is almost $140,000. In 1993, the total cost of cardiovascular disease in the United States reached $117.4 billion—and hypertension was a major contributor to its occurrence. In 2000, this cost has risen to $326 billion.

Most distressing is the fact that 30% of all hypertensive individuals are unaware that they have this condition. Only 70% of those diagnosed as hypertensives currently receive treatment, and only 27% of the 50 million people with this condition have their blood pressure properly controlled!

The good news is that hypertension can almost always be controlled and its complications minimized or prevented in the vast majority of people through appropriate therapy. During the past 25 years, the incidences of fatal strokes and fatal heart attacks have decreased by 60% and 53%, respectively. These remarkable results can be attributed to improved medical management of hypertension as well as healthy lifestyle changes in the United States.

The importance of a close patient–doctor relationship in the management of hypertension cannot be overemphasized. Optimal management of high blood pressure (hypertension) depends, to a large extent, on a clear appreciation of the risks of hypertension and an understanding of the appropriate treatment needed to prevent or minimize the occurrence of stroke, heart attack, heart and kidney failure, visual impairment, and hardening of the arteries. This fact inspired our 100 questions, some of which you may consider asking your physician. Ultimately, your knowledge about hypertension is key to ensuring successful treatment. You and your doctor should be *partners* in the management of your hypertension. The answers to the questions presented in this book provide important information that will better enable you to communicate with your doctor so that he or she may give you optimal care. Some of the answers are quite short, whereas others involve a detailed discussion.

We have attempted to answer each question thoroughly. As a result, considerable repetition occurs throughout the book. Answers to related questions are indicated in the text for the patient's convenience.

William M. Manger, MD, PhD
Ray W. Gifford, Jr., MD

Acknowledgments

It is hard to adequately thank our friends, patients, and colleagues who have contributed very helpful comments and suggestions regarding "100 Questions and Answers about Hypertension." We are especially grateful to the following whose constructive remarks have measurably improved the quality of this book.

Nelson Adams, Esq., Leslie Baer, MD, Ms. Henry Barbey, Ms. Florence Barbey, Mr. Henry Barbey III, George Beuttell, Henry Black, MD, Ms. Julia Carter, Ms. Emily Casson, Ms. Julia Casson, Dean Aram Chobanian, MD, Richard Coburn, MD, DMD, JD, Honorable Walter Curley, Ms. Willie Mae Darrisaw, Ms. Isabelle Dayton, John Dayton, MD, Mr. Louis DiCerbo, Ms. Irene Herlihy, Ms. Jill Hobbs, Joseph Izzo, MD, Norman Kaplan, MD, Claude Lenfant, MD, Ms. Lilian Lewis, Joseph Loscalzo, MD, Ms. Ann MacRae, Ms. Carol Manger, Charles Manger III, MD, Mr. Charles Manger IV, Ms. Holly Manger, Ms. Janice Manger, Jules Manger, MD, Mr. Jules Manger, Ms. Laurie Manger, Philip Manger, MD, Alexander Minno, MD, Francis Minno, Esq., Mr. Ray O'Connor, Ms. Irvine Page, Thomas Pickering, MD, Ed Roccella, PhD, MPH, Ms. Francine Rowley, Mr. Henry Rowley, Shlomoh Simchon, PhD, Ms. Sandra Stevens, Ms. Claire Van Zant, Peter Wall, Esq., Ms. Jean Waters, Ms. Erin Whitehead.

Very special thanks go to Ms. Ruth Johnston and Ms. Alla Krayko for their remarkable skill in proofreading and preparing this book.

Introduction

A broad need exists for increasing public and patient education regarding the problem of high blood pressure or hypertension. It is a highly prevalent clinical problem that afflicts more then 50 million adults in the United States. Its prevalence increases steadily with age so that more than 60% of men and women over age 65 have elevated levels of blood pressure, and as the population continues to increase in age, so will the number of individuals with hypertension. At any age, the higher the blood pressure, the greater the cardiovascular risks from hypertension including heart attacks, heart failure, angina, stroke, and kidney diseases. High blood pressure ranks in importance with abnormal blood cholesterol levels and smoking as major risk factors for cardiovascular diseases, and it augments even further the adverse effects of other such risk factors on these major causes of death and disability in our population.

Even modest increases in blood pressure can be detrimental to the cardiovascular system, and small reductions of blood pressure in the population as a whole, particularly in those with so-called "high normal levels" would be expected to have significant benefits. Lifestyle changes, non-drug approaches such as weight reduction, increased physical activity, and dietary changes that favor reduction in salt or sodium chloride and increase in foods that are high in potassium, grains, fruits, vegetables, and non-fat dairy products all may be of value. Obesity is not only a cause of hypertension but also contributes to abnormal blood fats and diabetes. Unfortunately, the prevalence of obesity has continued to increase significantly during the past decade.

Advances in drug therapy during the past half century have had a major impact on the ability to control hypertension. Several classes of effective medications have been introduced, and the capability now exists to normalize blood pressure in most hypertensive individuals. In addition, many clinical trials have confirmed the major benefits of the treatment of hypertension in reducing the most serious cardiovascular complications. Despite these well-known benefits, control of hypertension, even in affluent countries such as ours, is grossly inadequate. Various factors may be responsible for the poor control. Inadequate attention of physicians to management undoubtedly contributes to the problem. Failure of patients to adhere to prescribed therapy also plays an important role. Increased education of both groups will be required before improved control of hypertension is achieved.

As hypertension is a chronic disease which generally requires long-term therapy, any given hypertensive patient is likely to receive many different medications during his or her lifetime. These may vary in their mechanism of action and have different beneficial or adverse effects. Many of the patients also may use nature foods and other unapproved "alternative" medications to manage their hypertension. The diverse nature of these therapies and the various contributing causes of hypertension have served to create an environment that has bred many misconceptions and myths about the disease.

Several quality publications exist for public and patient education relating to hypertension and cardiovascular diseases. None of these, in my opinion, has utilized so effectively the question/answer approach that has been achieved by Drs. Manger and Gifford in this book. Both are distinguished physicians who are leaders in the field of hypertension. Their answers to the commonly asked questions are presented clearly and comprehensively. The book represents an important addition to the field and is recommended for patients and others interested in knowing more about the disease. It also has value as a reference guide for healthcare providers who deal frequently with hypertensive patients.

Aram Chobanian, MD
Dean and Provost, Medical Campus
Boston University School of Medicine

Notice: The indications and dosages of all drugs in this book have been recommended in the medical literature and conform to the practices followed by the general medical community. The medications described and treatment prescriptions suggested do not necessarily have specific approval by the U.S. Food and Drug Administration (FDA) for use in the diseases and dosages for which they are recommended. The package insert for each drug should be consulted to learn the use and dosage as approved by the FDA. Because standards for usage change, it is advisable to keep abreast of revised recommendations, particularly those concerning new drugs.

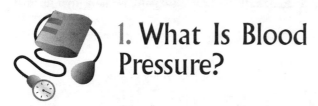

1. What Is Blood Pressure?

Blood pressure is the pressure exerted by the blood on the walls of the arteries. It depends on the amount of blood pumped by the heart and the resistance, which is caused mainly by the degree of constriction of the smallest arteries called arterioles. These arterioles have smooth muscle in their walls that can contract or relax, thereby altering the caliber of these vessels. Constriction of these vessels and increasing resistance to flow can raise pressure—the effect has been likened to bending a garden hose into a V shape or reducing the opening at the hose's nozzle to impede the flow of water and thus elevating the pressure of water in the hose. Pressure in the hose can also be increased by increasing the amount of water flowing from the faucet; this effect is analogous to the increased blood flow that ensues when the pumping action of the heart is augmented.

Blood pressure is the pressure exerted by the blood on the walls of the arteries.

Blood pressure varies considerably in everyone during the day, depending on the demands of the body. For example, blood pressure may increase markedly during exercise, when muscles require a greater supply of oxygen and nutrition. This elevated blood pressure results from an increased rate and pumping action of the heart; the arterioles in the muscles actually dilate to permit an increased blood supply. Similarly, anxiety during the "fight or flight" response can activate the sympathetic nervous system and cause liberation of adrenaline and similar hormones; as a result, the heart speeds up and pumps out more blood even as the arterioles become constricted, thereby increasing blood pressure.

During sleep, inactivity reduces the demand for oxygen. The rate and pumping action of the heart therefore decrease and the arterioles dilate. As a result, the blood pressure decreases. Normally, pressure is lowest at night and highest in the morning when arousal activates the sympathetic nervous system. Although blood pressure remains primarily under the control of the nervous system, a variety of substances and hormones released from the kidneys, heart, adrenal glands, and the lining of the blood vessels can play important roles in altering the caliber of the arterioles and can elevate or lower blood pressure in response to a variety of stressful conditions. Under normal circumstances, the arterioles are

1

relatively relaxed and dilated, and the blood pressure remains in a normal range.

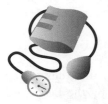

2. What Are Systolic, Diastolic, and Pulse Pressures?

Blood pressure (BP) is the force that blood exerts on the walls of the arteries as a result of the pumping action of the heart. It is determined by the amount of blood that the heart pumps every beat as well as by the resistance that the blood meets in the tiny microscopic blood vessels called arterioles. Anything that tends to constrict or narrow the arterioles will raise BP; conversely, anything that relaxes them will lower BP. An increase in the amount of blood that is pumped by the heart will not necessarily increase BP if the arterioles dilate to lessen the resistance that the blood meets.

Systolic BP is the pressure generated by each beat of the heart; it is so named because each beat or contraction of the heart is known as a "systole." **Diastolic BP is the pressure between heart beats**, when the heart is not contracting; this event is known as a "diastole." Systolic BP is always higher than diastolic BP because it is generated by the force of the heart beat. BP is usually expressed as systolic BP over diastolic BP in millimeters of mercury (for example, 130/80 mm Hg). Pulse pressure is the difference between systolic and diastolic BP. For example, when the systolic pressure is 130 mm Hg and the diastolic pressure is 80 mm Hg (130/80 mm Hg), the pulse pressure is 50 (130 − 80 = 50). Significant elevation of any of these pressures increases the risk of heart disease, stroke, and kidney disease.

Pulse pressure is the difference between systolic and diastolic BP.

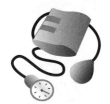

3. How Is Blood Pressure Measured?

Blood pressure in the doctor's office is usually measured with a stethoscope and a sphygmomanometer (Figure 1). The latter instrument contains a glass tube in which the height of a mercury column indicates the

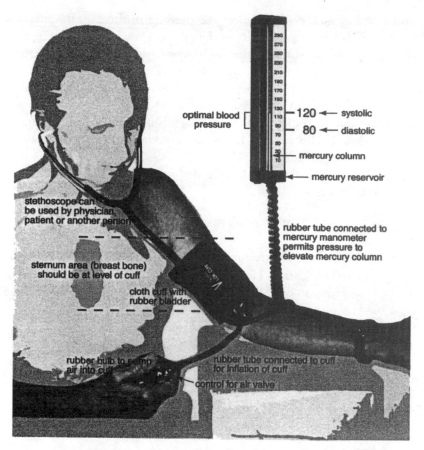

optimal blood pressure

120 ← systolic
80 ← diastolic

mercury column

mercury reservoir

rubber tube connected to mercury manometer permits pressure to elevate mercury column

stethoscope can be used by physician patient or another person

sternum area (breast bone) should be at level of cuff

cloth cuff with rubber bladder

rubber bulb to pump air into cuff

rubber tube connected to cuff for inflation of cuff

control for air valve

Figure 1. **Patient Measuring Blood Pressure in Arm with Sphygmomanometer and Stethoscope**

pressure. Measuring blood pressure is quite simple and requires very little training.

The sphygmomanometer consists of a cloth cuff containing an inflatable rubber bag, which is connected by a rubber tube to a reservoir of mercury. The cuff is wrapped around the patient's upper arm, with the lower edge remaining approximately one inch above the arm crease. Repeatedly squeezing a rubber bulb pumps air through another tube into the rubber bag. The pressure in the bag, which is the same as that elevating the column of mercury, increases until it temporarily occludes the flow of blood in the arm. At this point, the listening device of a stethoscope is placed over the inner side of the elbow crease, just below the cuff. When blood flow is occluded, no sound is heard with the stethoscope. Air is then gradually released through a valve in the

Blood pressure in the doctor's office is usually measured with a stethoscope and a sphygmomanometer.

rubber bulb, which slowly reduces the pressure in the bag; the mercury column will fall at the same time. At the moment at which the first thumping sound is heard through the stethoscope, the level of the mercury column in millimeters is recorded as the systolic pressure; it indicates the pressure when the heart is contracting and blood begins to flow through the arm. As the pressure in the bag continues to fall, the thumping sounds (which are due to spurts of blood with each heart contraction) can no longer be heard. This point is recorded in millimeters of mercury as the diastolic pressure (Figure 2).

Blood pressure is stated as systolic BP over diastolic BP and recorded with two numbers as follows:

$$\frac{\text{Systolic}}{\text{Diastolic}} \ \text{mm Hg (millimeters of mercury)}$$

Normal systolic pressures for adults more than 18 years old usually range from 100 to 130 mm Hg and diastolic pressures from 60 to 85 mm Hg. Systolic pressures of 130 to 139 mm Hg and diastolic pressures of 85 to 89 mm Hg, formerly considered high normal, are now considered elevated. In general, persons with relatively low systolic and diastolic pressures are less likely to develop strokes, heart disease, or kidney disease (Figure 2).

Although other reliable sphygmomanometers are available for measuring blood pressure, their accuracy should be periodically compared

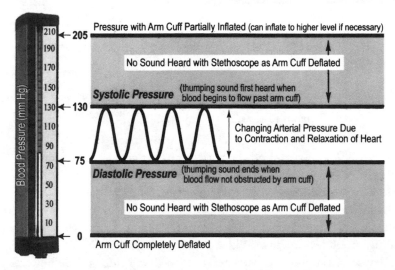

Figure 2. **Blood presure measurement in arm with sphygmomanometer and stethoscope**

with the results obtained via a sphygmomanometer that uses a mercury column, as the latter instrument is the most accurate. One popular and convenient device for measuring blood pressure is the aneroid sphygmomanometer, whose gauge indicates blood pressure by measuring the tension on a spring instead of the height of a mercury column; a stethoscope is still required, however. Electronic sphygmomanometers with a digital display of the blood pressure and pulse rate are especially convenient, because they do not require a stethoscope. We recommend the use of such instruments with an arm cuff, as the finger and wrist cuffs are usually less accurate. Electronic sphygmomanometers have an especially desirable feature—the rubber bag in the cuff can be automatically inflated and deflated by simply pressing a button. (The Omron HEM-704C, Omron 705CP and X, and Sunbeam 7650 self-inflating sphygmomanometers have been reported to be quite accurate.)

Blood pressure should be determined in either arm when the patient is in the seated position, because the risks of elevated blood pressure have been determined based on studies of blood pressures taken while in the seated posture. Blood pressure will be the same in both arms unless the patient has a rare vascular abnormality or some other condition that compresses the circulation to one arm and not the other. Additional information may be obtained by measuring blood pressure in the recumbent and standing positions, as these data may help establish whether blood pressure is normal in these positions and whether treatment is effective.

It is especially important that the person remains seated and resting in a quiet environment for at least five minutes before blood pressure measurements are taken. Cigarette smoking, consumption of drinks containing caffeine, and exercise should be avoided for approximately one hour before the blood pressure is measured. Crossing the legs and even just talking can elevate blood pressure. It is also important that the arm cuff be at the level of the heart (that is, the level of the breast bone) and that the proper size cuff be used, which depends on the size of the arm.

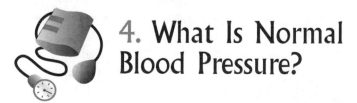

4. What Is Normal Blood Pressure?

For many years, 140/90 mm Hg was considered the dividing line between normal and high blood pressure (or at least it was widely accepted as the upper limit for which life insurance would be issued). Observational studies have since shown conclusively that risk begins with any systolic blood pressure exceeding 120 mm Hg and any diastolic blood pressure exceeding 80 mm Hg. The fifth and sixth reports of the Joint National Committee on the Prevention, Detection, Evaluation, and Treatment of High Blood Pressure (JNC V and JNC VI) desig-

Optimal blood pressure is 120/80 mm Hg or less, normal blood pressure is less than 130/80 mm Hg, and high-normal pressure is 130–139/85–89 mm Hg.

nated optimal blood pressure as 120/80 mm Hg or less, normal blood pressure as less than 130/80 mm Hg, and high-normal pressure as 130–139/85–89 mm Hg.

It should be realized that one determination of blood pressure may not be representative of the usual blood pressure—particularly if the reading is high. For this reason, most physicians do not initiate treatment on the basis of a single elevated blood pressure reading unless it is extremely high or unless the patient already has some evidence of "target organ disease" (such as damage to the heart, brain, kidneys, or eyes) or additional risk factors. Such risk factors may include elevated "bad" cholesterol [low-density lipoprotein (LDL) cholesterol] or triglyceride levels in the blood, cigarette smoking, diabetes mellitus, sedentary lifestyle, or a family history of premature heart attack or stroke in a parent or sibling.

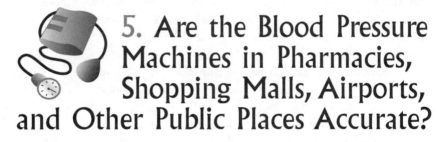

5. Are the Blood Pressure Machines in Pharmacies, Shopping Malls, Airports, and Other Public Places Accurate?

The blood pressure machines found in public places may be accurate, if properly used, when they are first installed. Like any apparatus for measuring blood pressure, however, they must be checked (calibrated) frequently, especially if they are used often, to maintain accuracy. Unless you know for certain that such devices are serviced regularly, it is hardly worth the effort to use them because of the aggravation that an erroneous reading may produce.

The blood pressure machines found in public places may be accurate, if properly used, but must be checked (calibrated) frequently to maintain that accuracy.

It is important to remember that, to ensure the most accurate blood pressure recordings, the individual should be seated and at rest for at least five minutes before the pressure is measured (see Question 3). If others are waiting to use the sphygmomanometer in a busy public area, a five-minute period of rest before pressure determination may not be possible. Just the stress of being in a rush to take the reading, talking, or holding a heavy package may raise blood pressure significantly. In addition, cigarette smoking, exercise, and caffeine consumption should be avoided for one hour or more before attempting such a measurement. If the blood pressure is elevated, the measurement should be repeated one or two more times to see whether it decreases with time and relaxation. Of course, multiple determinations may not be practical in a busy shopping center.

For hypertensive patients who want to monitor their blood pressure between doctor visits, we suggest purchasing a sphygmomanometer (with a cuff that is applied to the upper arm) from a pharmacy or medical supply store and then using that instrument in your home. Most physicians' office staff will be more than happy to show you how to use it properly and will tell you how often to take such measurements. Patients should keep a record of their blood pressures to show their doctors at subsequent visits.

The "Cadillac" of sphygmomanometers—which automatically inflates and deflates the cuff and gives a digital readout of blood pressure and pulse rate, sometimes with a slip of paper indicating the date and time of the recording—will cost more than $100. Ideally, the patient should not have to inflate the cuff by repeatedly compressing a rubber bulb, as this activity may raise the blood pressure slightly.

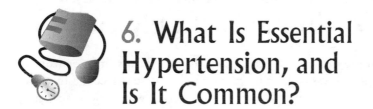

6. What Is Essential Hypertension, and Is It Common?

Essential (primary) hypertension is by far the most common type of hypertension. After your doctor excludes the causes of secondary hypertension (about 5% of hypertensives), which can be identified and often corrected (see Question 38), the vast majority of patients are found to have "essential" hypertension (about 95% of all hypertensives). This term is a misnomer because primary hypertension is not essential for anything! National health surveys suggest that more than 50 million Americans (25% of all adults) have systolic blood pressures of 140 mm Hg or higher and diastolic blood pressures of 90 mm Hg or higher. This condition is more common in elderly people and in African Americans. For example, more than 60% of African American women who are older than age 60 are believed to have hypertension.

Although the precise cause of essential hypertension remains unknown, this condition is probably the result of multiple factors (see Questions 11, 13, 33). Heredity certainly plays a role in most cases, and more than one genetic abnormality seems to exist. In addition, environmental factors can contribute to the development of hypertension. Some individuals are salt-sensitive, and excess salt consumption will elevate their blood pressure. Being overweight or obese, consuming excessive amounts of alcohol, following a sedentary lifestyle, and eating a low-potassium diet may also elevate blood pressure in persons with essential hypertension. Although you can't change your genes, gender, age, or racial background, you can certainly avoid environmental factors that may cause or aggravate hypertension. It is noteworthy that healthy lifestyle modifications may not only reduce elevated blood pressure, but also prevent hypertension in a significant segment of the population.

The cause or causes of essential hypertension are unknown but both heredity and environmental factors such as salt sensitivity, obesity, consumption of excessive amounts of alcohol, a sedentary lifestyle, and a diet low in potassium can play a role in its development and severity.

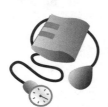

7. Why Is High Blood Pressure Bad, and Does Treatment Really Help?

Long ago, insurance companies learned that applicants (men or women) with high blood pressure have more strokes, heart attacks, congestive heart failure, kidney failure, and diseases of the arteries, which more frequently lead to disability or premature death, than do applicants with "normal" blood pressures. This fact explains why you cannot get life or disability insurance at standard rates if you have hypertension.

Patients whose blood pressure is lowered with medication have less risk of stroke, heart attack, and heart failure as well as a prolonged useful life as compared with patients who are given placebos.

Numerous clinical trials have clearly proved that patients whose blood pressure is lowered with medication have less risk of stroke, heart attack, and heart failure as well as a prolonged useful life as compared with patients who are given placebos (see Question 74). In fact, these studies have yielded such convincing results that it is now considered unethical to use placebos in trials for more than a short time in almost all patients with hypertension. The ability of newer drugs to control blood pressure and prevent complications must now be compared to the activity of older or standard medications (rather than placebos) in trials designed to evaluate their effectiveness.

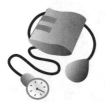 # 8. What Is the Magnitude of the Hypertension Problem in the United States?

- **Hypertension, along with its complications (stroke, heart attack, heart failure, and kidney failure), is the leading cause of death in the United States, killing almost 1 million people each year.** This condition accelerates hardening of the arteries. Other conditions (such as cigarette smoking, abnormal blood lipids, diabetes, obesity, and sedentary lifestyle) can also contribute to the complications of hypertension (see Question 43).

- In the United States, 50 million adults have hypertension—defined as sustained elevations of blood pressure above 140 mm Hg systolic and/or 90 mm Hg diastolic. Almost one of every four adult Americans has hypertension.

- Of the 50 million Americans with hypertension, 32% are unaware that they have this condition. Only 78% of diagnosed patients receive treatment—so 27 million individuals with hypertension receive no treatment at all.

- Only 27% of the 50 million Americans with hypertension have their blood pressure under control. Thus more than 36 million people have uncontrolled hypertension.

- Hypertension is the most important cause of invalidism and lost productivity because of brain, heart, and kidney damage. It cripples and disables almost 1 million people each year and is the most common reason for visiting a doctor's office.

- One of every five persons in the work force has high blood pressure. One-half of all hypertensives are in the work force. Hypertension, with its complications of stroke and heart attack, is responsible for 52 million workdays of lost productivity for business.

- In 1991 in the United States, cardiovascular disease and stroke were responsible for nearly 4 million years of life lost before reaching the age of 75.

- In 2000, the total cost of cardiovascular disease in the United States will reach an estimated $326 billion, with hypertension being a very important contributor to this expense.

- More than 75% of stroke victims have high blood pressure. Strokes cost Americans $45 billion in medical bills and lost earnings each year. The average lifetime cost to the patient who suffers a nonfatal stroke is almost $140,000.

- Hypertension develops earlier and generally becomes more severe in African Americans than it is in Caucasians. Stroke and heart disease mortality are 80% and 50% greater, respectively, and severe hypertensive kidney disease occurs 320% more often in African Americans than they do in Caucasians.

- **Treatment of hypertension saves lives and prevents disability!**

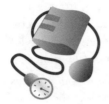

9. What Are Some Common Misconceptions About Hypertension?

Many members of the public hold a number of misconceptions or myths relating to high blood pressure. Such misinformation deserves correction and clarification, because it can interfere with the proper management of individuals with hypertension. The more common and prevalent misconceptions follow.

1. **Many persons with hypertension are convinced that they can tell by the way they feel whether their blood pressure is elevated.** Experience with blood pressure determinations by professionals or by individuals with hypertension or with 24-hour monitoring devices has shown that patients are usually unable to detect when their blood pressure is high. On the other hand, pain, stress, anxiety, and fear may significantly increase blood pressure in most people, regardless of whether they are hypertensive. In addition, some people have "white-coat hypertension" (see Question 14). Under these circumstances, the individual is aware of emotional tension and may correctly guess that blood pressure is elevated, even though no sensation specifically alerts the individual that the pressure is elevated. Feeling very well has nothing to do with blood pressure level and is never an indication that antihypertensive medication should be discontinued.

2. **Some people believe that systolic blood pressure should be roughly 100 plus your age, and that blood pressure becomes elevated to maintain adequate flow to the organs of the body.** Essential hypertension is the most common form of hypertension [accounting for roughly 95% of all cases of elevated blood pressure (see Question 6)]. In this condition, usually both the systolic (the top number) and diastolic (the bottom number) pressures are elevated. Most such cases appear in midlife (35 to 50 years of age).

   On the other hand, elevation of the systolic pressure does tend to occur in industrialized countries, where most people consume diets that can increase weight and lead to obesity, hardening of the arteries, and hypertension. This higher systolic pressure results from the loss of elasticity of the aorta—the largest artery in the body, which directly receives blood pumped from the heart. As the aorta hardens (becomes arteriosclerotic), its elasticity (its ability to expand when the heart pumps blood into it) progressively diminishes with aging. As a result, the blood expelled with each contraction (systole) of the heart meets increased resistance because of rigidity in the aorta, and the systolic blood pressure becomes progressively elevated. In primitive societies, where people are not sedentary and consume little fat, dairy products, or salt, blood pressure and body weight do not become elevated with aging. Clearly, then, aging alone does not increase blood pressure. Instead, stiffness of the aorta results largely from poor dietary habits, lack of exercise, and weight gain.

   Hypertension never results from the body's efforts to improve the circulation of various organs; rather, it reflects an abnormal increase of resistance in large arteries due to atherosclerosis and constriction of small arteries (arterioles). As we all know, hypertension can lead to many complications (including heart attack, stroke, heart and kidney failure, hardening of arteries, and very rarely visual impairment). Conversely, lowering blood pressure can prevent or minimize these complications.

3. **Many persons believe that hypertension indicates that a person is too tense because of excess stress** (see Question 23). In reality, hypertension simply means high blood pressure. There is no proof that individuals who feel chronically tense and nervous have higher blood pressures than those who feel calm and relaxed. Of course, sudden fright, fear, or anxiety can evoke the "fight or flight" response with its ensuing release of adrenaline and activation of the sympathetic nervous system; this response can cause constriction of arteries, which elevates

blood pressure. Nevertheless, this natural and temporary response does not result in sustained hypertension.

Very significant elevations of blood pressure are encountered in approximately 20% of all nonhypertensive individuals when their blood pressure is measured by a doctor. This phenomenon is known as "white-coat hypertension," because the doctor is perceived as a possible bearer of bad news. Again, no strong evidence exists to show that most of these individuals, whose blood pressures are usually normal at other times, are prone to developing sustained hypertension and therefore require prophylactic antihypertensive medication. On the other hand, no strong evidence indicates that many of these patients will not eventually become hypertensive. Consequently, the blood pressures of individuals with "white-coat hypertension" (see Question 14) should be checked more frequently than those of normal subjects to identify anyone who might develop sustained hypertension.

4. **Some persons believe that they can always control their blood pressures with lifestyle changes.** Although reduction of excess weight, limitation of excess consumption of dietary salt and alcohol, consumption of a diet with lots of fruits and vegetables and little saturated fat, and adequate exercise may sometimes normalize mild or even moderately elevated blood pressure, antihypertensive medication is usually required to realize optimal blood pressure control. If blood pressure is severely elevated (180/110 mm Hg or greater), antihypertensive drugs are almost always necessary to achieve optimal control (that is, blood pressures of 130/80 mm Hg or less). Antihypertensive medication is most effective, and smaller doses are often required, in persons closely adhering to the lifestyle changes mentioned above. Only rarely can antihypertensive medication be discontinued, although with appropriate lifestyle changes—especially considerable weight loss in obese individuals—it may be possible to reduce or discontinue medication. (See Question 55.)

5. **Some persons with hypertension believe that they have to limit their activities.** It is prudent for patients with very severe hypertension to initially avoid very strenuous exercise, especially weightlifting, as this activity can temporarily elevate blood pressure to dangerous levels. Regular exercise (brisk walking for approximately three hours each week is excellent) is strongly recommended (see Question 46), however, provided that appropriate testing has ruled out the presence of heart disease that might result in heart failure, a heart attack, or serious arrhythmia (irregularity of the heart rhythm). Also, complications of hypertension—such as stroke, kidney failure, an aortic aneurysm (a weakness with bulging of a portion of the aorta), or decreased blood supply to

the legs because of atherosclerosis—may, of course, curtail activity. If the individual does not suffer from any of these complications, proper control of blood pressure with antihypertensive drugs and lifestyle changes should permit the hypertensive patient to lead a perfectly normal life without curtailing any routine activities.

6. **Many persons, including some physicians, believe that the elderly (a) comply poorly when taking their medication, (b) do not tolerate their medication very well, and (c) will not benefit much from taking antihypertensive drugs.** All of these theories about the elderly have been proved wrong. In fact, older persons take their medication as well, if not better, than younger patients, and treatment is particularly beneficial in the elderly. Smaller doses of medication may be indicated in some older patients, particularly in thin and frail individuals. Nevertheless, with appropriate dosage schedules, elderly patients tolerate medications as well as their younger counterparts.

7. **Most laypersons and many physicians believe that the level of the diastolic blood pressure is far more important than the level of the systolic pressure as a risk for heart attack and stroke.** This concept was previously accepted and widely taught in medical schools. More recently, it has become abundantly clear that the reverse is true—lowering *systolic* pressure is crucial to the prevention of cardiovascular disease and stroke!

8. **Some patients believe that they can stop taking their antihypertensive medicine when their hypertension is brought under control.** Treatment of hypertension merely controls this condition, but does not cure it. When your doctor tells you that your blood pressure is well controlled, it doesn't mean that you can stop the medicine—it means that you must continue to take it if you want to keep your blood pressure at a healthy level.

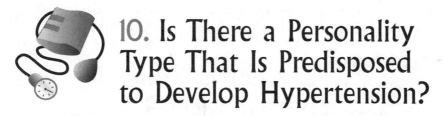

10. Is There a Personality Type That Is Predisposed to Develop Hypertension?

No particular personality type is more likely to develop hypertension. Some psychologists and psychiatrists identify the "hypertensive personality" as rigid, compulsive, and occurring in an individual who cannot openly express hostility. It has been suggested that persons with type A personalities—that is, those who are particularly competitive, aggressive, ambitious, and hard-driving—may activate their sympathetic nervous systems, thereby constricting their arteries and causing hypertension and coronary heart disease. In reality, most hypertensive patients do not have these personality traits or, if they do, it takes a psychiatrist or psychologist to find them! Many hypertensive patients are relaxed, phlegmatic, and indifferent. No personality type is immune to the threat of hypertension, and no strong evidence proves that subjects with type A personalities are more likely to develop hypertension than any others.

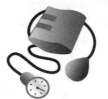

11. Is Essential (Primary) Hypertension Inherited?

Essential hypertension is inherited or at least frequently runs in families—but so do other unhealthy characteristics and lifestyles (such as obesity,

Essential hypertension is inherited or at least frequently runs in families—but so do other unhealthy characteristics and lifestyles.

exercise involvement, alcohol consumption, and dietary habits). Blood pressure usually increases with increasing weight, and almost 50% of obese people have high blood pressure. If one parent has essential hypertension, his or her child has a 25% chance of developing hypertension; this risk increases to approximately 75% if both parents are hypertensive.

Much research is now devoted to identifying genes that might cause high blood pressure. Eventually, multiple genes will probably be implicated because it is unlikely that all patients with hypertension share the same genetic abnormalities. For example, as many as 60% of all hypertensive individuals are salt-sensitive—but the other 40% are not. Furthermore, the incidence of hypertension among African Americans may be at least twice that observed among whites. Clearly, the cause of essential hypertension is complex and influenced by multiple factors (see Question 6).

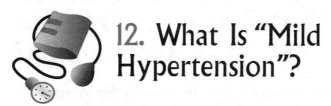

12. What Is "Mild Hypertension"?

The term "mild hypertension" was discarded by the Fifth and Sixth Joint National Committees on the Prevention, Detection, Evaluation, and

Table 1. *Classification of Blood Pressure for Adults Age 18 and Older**

Category	Systolic (mm Hg)		Diastolic (mm Hg)
Optimal†	<120	and	<80
Normal	<130	and	<85
High normal	130–139	or	85–89
Hypertension‡			
Stage 1	140–159	or	90–99
Stage 2	160–179	or	100–109
Stage 3	≥180	or	≥110

* Not taking antihypertensive drugs and not acutely ill. Isolated systolic hypertension is defined as systolic BP of 140 mm Hg or greater and diastolic BP of less than 90 mm Hg. In addition to classifying stages of hypertension on the basis of average blood pressure levels, clinicians should indicate the presence or absence of target organ disease and additional risk factors. This information is important for risk classification and treatment.

† Optimal blood pressure with respect to cardiovascular risk is less than 120/80 mm Hg, but unusually low readings should be evaluated for clinical significance.

‡ Based on the average of two or more readings taken at each of two or more visits after an initial screening.

Treatment of High Blood Pressure (JNC V and JNC VI) because it is misleading. While it is true that the higher the blood pressure, the greater the risk of complications, even patients with "mild" hypertension" (systolic blood pressures in the vicinity of 140 mm Hg and diastolic pressures near 90 mm Hg) are at increased risk of having a stroke, heart attack, heart failure, or kidney failure, although those events may take longer to happen. The JNC V and JNC VI reports have recommended using "stages" of hypertension, rather than the old terminology of "mild," "moderate," and "severe" (Table 1). Optimal, normal, and high-normal blood pressures are also included in Table 1.

> *The term "mild hypertension" has been largely discarded because it is misleading.*

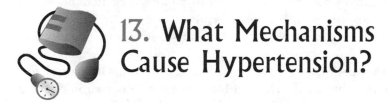

13. What Mechanisms Cause Hypertension?

Blood pressure is dependent on the heart rate, the amount of blood pumped with each beat, and the degree of constriction in the arterioles. Other factors, such as the amount of blood in the circulation and even the thickness of the blood (which largely depends on the number of red blood cells in the circulation), can also influence the blood pressure.

It is important to understand that blood pressure may vary considerably during the day and that it can be influenced by many conditions. Conditions that increase the pumping action of the heart—such as exercise, some drugs and hormones, or increased blood volume—can increase the amount of blood pumped with each heart beat and hence elevate blood pressure, particularly the systolic pressure (which occurs during contraction of the heart). Hardening of the large arteries (arteriosclerosis) of the body may also increase systolic pressure.

Conditions that increase the pumping action of the heart can increase the amount of blood pumped with each heart beat and hence elevate blood pressure, particularly the systolic pressure. Conditions that activate the sympathetic nervous system and stimulate vascular smooth muscles cause constriction of arterioles and also elevate blood pressure, primarily the diastolic pressure.

On the other hand, conditions that activate the sympathetic nervous system—such as stimulation of the nervous system, neurohormones, certain drugs, emotional tension, and severe cold—and stimulate vascular smooth muscles promote constriction of arterioles. This constriction also elevates blood pressure, primarily the diastolic pressure (the pressure when the heart is not contracting, which mainly depends on the degree of constriction of the arterioles).

Occasionally, with sudden fear and anxiety (the "fight or flight" reaction), increased pumping action of the heart and constriction of arterioles may occur together and boost blood pressure. Even normal individuals periodically have hypertensive blood pressure elevations during the day (see Question 36). These transitory elevations pose no serious risk.

Essential or primary hypertension, which accounts for 95% of all hypertension cases, exists when elevations in blood pressure are sustained without any obvious cause. Genetics can certainly play a role in this condition's development, as the condition is much more common in the offspring of parents who have hypertension; multiple hypertension-related genetic abnormalities appear to exist. Furthermore, perhaps 60% of persons with essential hypertension are salt-sensitive; that is, excess salt consumption causes hypertension in these individuals (see Question 34). Exactly why salt produces hypertension remains unclear. **The main abnormality responsible for the elevated blood pressure observed in essential hypertension appears to be increased constriction of the arterioles, but the cause of this constriction remains unknown.**

The causes of secondary hypertension, which account for only 5% of all hypertensive patients, are known and are discussed in detail in Question 38. They relate to damaged kidneys or functional impairment, hormonal tumors, and other endocrine abnormalities. In particular, a variety of drugs and hormones, some conditions that stimulate the nervous system, preeclampsia or eclampsia during pregnancy, coarctation (constriction) of the aorta, and sleep apnea can cause hypertension. In these conditions, the hypertension may result from increased constriction of arterioles, increased pumping action of the heart, or both. The hypertension in coarctation, which occurs only in the upper part of the body, is mainly due to the blockage of blood flow caused by the coarctation; impaired blood flow to the kidneys resulting from the coarctation may, however, also produce a substance that constricts arterioles.

Hypertension is, therefore, a manifestation of an increased resistance to blood flow because of constriction of arterioles or occasionally an increased output of blood by the heart, or a combination of these changes. As indicated above, a large number of conditions and diseases may be responsible for these changes that produce hypertension.

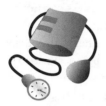 14. What Is "White-Coat Hypertension"? Do I Have It and Is It Dangerous?

"White-coat hypertension" is hypertension that occurs only when blood pressure is taken by the doctor; in this condition, blood pressure remains normal when measured by the patient or by others at home, in the workplace, or elsewhere (see Question 19). According to Dr. Tom Pickering, a specialist in hypertension, who has extensively studied this type of hypertension, 20% of patients who have diastolic pressures between 90 and 100 mm Hg when measured by the doctor in his or her office subsequently demonstrate normal blood pressures when they are automatically monitored for 24 hours.

> *"White-coat hypertension" is hypertension that occurs only when blood pressure is taken by the doctor; blood pressure remains normal when measured by the patient or by others at home, in the workplace, or elsewhere.*

Although white-coat hypertension may affect anyone, it is slightly more common in women than in men. It occurs in approximately 40% of all individuals older than age 65 when blood pressure is determined by the doctor. No evidence suggests that persons with white-coat hypertension have a certain type of personality or are more neurotic than anyone else; furthermore, their blood pressures react to a variety of stresses in the same way as do the blood pressures of individuals without white-coat hypertension. It appears that the doctor (the "white-coat" figure) engenders a significant sense of fear and anxiety in certain patients, sometimes even accompanied by an increase in heart rate, which results in an abnormal increase in blood pressure. This reaction probably reflects some apprehension that the doctor may report bad news—that is, that the patient's blood pressure is elevated. This threat may persist for years when blood pressure is measured by the doctor, despite a prolonged and friendly relationship with the physician.

White-coat hypertension requires that the blood pressure be usually in the hypertensive range (greater than 140/90 mm Hg) when recorded by the doctor on several office visits, but consistently normal when recorded elsewhere. For accurate blood pressure determinations, it is important that the patient remains seated and relaxed in a quiet environment for at least five minutes; that the individual avoids exercise, smoking, and drinks containing caffeine for one hour before the recording, and that the patient avoids stress of any type just prior to the measurement. Chronic excess consumption of alcohol may also increase blood pressure. Blood pressure may be taken frequently throughout the day by the patient or other individuals or it may be monitored every 15 minutes and recorded by an automatic electronic device. Machines to record blood pressures in pharmacies and shopping areas may not always be accurate, however (see Question 5).

Patients who are truly hypertensive will have elevated blood pressure no matter who takes the measurement and no matter where it is taken. Of course, hypertensive patients may also be apprehensive when the doctor measures their blood pressure and may have somewhat higher blood pressure in that circumstance than when pressure is measured by someone else, outside the doctor's office.

It remains unclear whether individuals with white-coat hypertension are more likely to develop sustained hypertension and its associated complications than are persons whose blood pressures remain less than 140/90 mm Hg, both inside and outside the doctor's office. It is not recommended that antihypertensive medication be given to persons with white-coat hypertension, if the condition has not damaged the heart, brain, or blood vessels elsewhere. However, blood pressures in persons with white-coat hypertension should be measured every few months to verify that persistent hypertension has not developed, as some evidence suggests that these patients have a greater chance of developing hypertension than normal subjects. Furthermore, it is recommended that patients with white-coat hypertension, if indicated, lose weight, stop smoking, limit salt and alcohol consumption, and undertake adequate aerobic exercise. Checking the blood pressure frequently—at least several times each year—

and making any necessary lifestyle changes will ensure the proper management of patients with this type of hypertension.

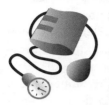

15. What Are the Purposes of the Pretreatment Examination?

There are four main reasons why patients with hypertension should be evaluated before starting treatment:

- To identify patients who have a curable cause for their high blood pressure.
- To assess the status of the organs targeted by hypertension—namely, the heart, brain, eyes, kidneys, and the blood vessels.
- To identify other cardiovascular risk factors—for example, diabetes, smoking, high serum cholesterol, age, upper body obesity, sedentary lifestyle, family history of premature stroke or heart attack—that could affect the need for and the choice of treatment.
- To ensure that the elevated blood pressure is sustained over a period of time—that is, to rule out "white-coat hypertension," which is caused by anxiety in the presence of the doctor (see Question 14).

The tests that a doctor may order to get this information are discussed in Question 16.

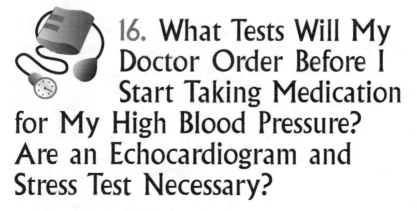

16. What Tests Will My Doctor Order Before I Start Taking Medication for My High Blood Pressure? Are an Echocardiogram and Stress Test Necessary?

Not everyone who has high blood pressure (hypertension) needs medication. The purpose of the examination is to aid the physician in deciding whether you need only medication, only lifestyle changes, or a combination of the two. For patients with Stage 1 hypertension (Table 2; also see Question 12), no evidence of target organ disease (that is, no apparent heart, brain, kidney, or visual damage), and no other risk factors (such as cigarette smoking, blood lipid abnormalities, diabetes, obesity, or sedentary lifestyle), medication might be appropriately withheld until the full benefits of lifestyle modifications can be achieved.

The purpose of the examination is to aid the physician in deciding whether you need only medication, only lifestyle changes, or a combination of the two.

Usually an electrocardiogram is recommended to evaluate the heart. Blood tests help rule out diabetes mellitus; they evaluate your cholesterol levels, including levels of LDL (low-density lipoprotein, or "bad" cholesterol) and HDL (high-density lipoprotein, or "good" cholesterol), as well as your triglyceride level (another type of lipid)—that is, fats that may damage blood vessels and cause heart disease. Multiple determinations of blood pressure both in the office and sometimes in your home are necessary to establish a baseline and to exclude the possibility of "white-coat hypertension" (see Question 14) before any treatment is prescribed. A physical examination is also important to identify target organ disease or curable secondary causes of high blood pressure. In addition, a urinalysis is helpful to evaluate the kidney as a target organ. All of this information aids your physician in determining appropriate treatment.

An echocardiogram is usually not necessary. The electrocardiogram, which reveals the electrical activity of the heart, is much simpler to perform, much less expensive, and it usually provides the information needed for evaluating the heart prior to treatment. In some cases, and

Table 2. *Classification of Blood Pressure for Adults Age 18 Years and Older*

Category	Systolic (mm Hg)		Diastolic (mm Hg)
Optimal*	<120	and	<80
Normal	<130	and	<85
High normal	130–139	or	85–89
Hypertension			
Stage 1	140–159	or	90–99
Stage 2	160–179	or	100–109
Stage 3	≥180	or	≥110

*Optimal blood pressure with respect to cardiovascular risk is less than 120/80 mm Hg.
Source: Joint National Committee—VI Report (JNC VI).

especially when heart failure is suspected, an echocardiogram, which visualizes the size, configuration, and pumping action of the heart, provides more detailed information than the electrocardiogram. The echocardiogram is much more sensitive in detecting early evidence of enlargement and thickening of the walls of the heart. Enlargement of the heart sometimes accompanies hypertension and may require more aggressive treatment.

A chest X ray may be ordered, especially if the patient has not received one for many years, just to confirm that no abnormalities of the lungs or heart are present. If the patient has had hypertension for a long time, the X ray may reveal enlargement of the heart, especially the left ventricle. The left ventricle, which is the main pumping chamber of the heart, has to pump against the elevated pressure.

A stress test, in which the electrocardiogram is recorded during exercise, is not routinely ordered; however, if there is any suggestion of chest pressure sensations or pain that might be due to coronary artery disease, then a stress test is usually indicated. For men more than 45 years old and postmenopausal women, it is sometimes prudent to obtain a stress test to help detect impaired circulation to the heart, especially in those patients planning to begin an exercise program.

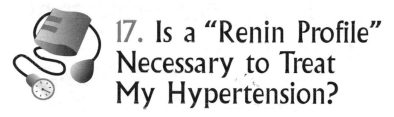

17. Is a "Renin Profile" Necessary to Treat My Hypertension?

A renin profile is not necessary to begin hypertension treatment. The renin profile measures an enzyme called renin in the blood. Physicians had hoped that the serum concentration of renin (which generates a hypertensive substance called angiotensin) would predict which medications would be the most appropriate and effective for a given patient. Generally, patients with low-renin hypertension respond well to diuretics whereas those with high-renin hypertension respond well to angiotensin-converting enzyme (ACE) inhibitors or angiotensin II (A II) blockers. Unfortunately, the renin profile has not proved to be a valuable therapeutic guide and is unnecessary and can even be misleading. Insurance companies will not pay for it either. In special circumstances, determination of the renin level in the blood may help identify patients in whom hypertension results from excess production of renin by the kidney.

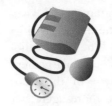

18. Do I Need to See a Specialist to Have My Hypertension Treated?

The vast majority of hypertensive patients are treated by family physicians who are knowledgeable about the variety of drugs available. The reasons for referral to a specialist might include the following:

- Difficulty in keeping your blood pressure controlled to less than 130/80 mm Hg most of the time without side effects from medication
- Complications of hypertension
- Multiple risk factors in addition to hypertension.

If a secondary cause of hypertension is suspected, consultation with a hypertension specialist may help establish the diagnosis and decide on the appropriate management tactics for the rarer causes of elevated blood pressure.

19. Are Measurements of Blood Pressure at Home Important in Managing Hypertension, and Should I Have My Blood Pressure Monitored for 24 Hours?

Although home blood pressure measurements can be extremely valuable in the management of hypertension, 24-hour monitoring of blood pressure by an electronic device is rarely necessary for diagnosis and treatment.

Without doubt, home blood pressure measurements can be extremely valuable in the management of hypertension (see Question 14). On the other hand, 24-hour monitoring of your blood pressure by an electronic device is rarely necessary for diagnosis and treatment. Such monitoring costs approximately $150 to $250, and is not reimbursable by most insurance companies.

Home blood pressure measurements offer two major advantages:

- They can establish whether elevated blood pressure in the doctor's office involves "white-coat hypertension" due to emotional tension from anxiety and fear (see Question 14).

- They enable your physician to evaluate the effectiveness of antihypertensive medications and to make appropriate adjustments in dosage.

In addition, the discipline required to keep records of home-measured blood pressures and periodically report these results can lead to a stronger patient–doctor relationship and help ensure that patients continue taking their medication. Finally, the need for office visits may be very significantly reduced, providing considerable savings to the patient in terms of medical expenses and the time and inconvenience of office visits.

Very few patients cannot measure their blood pressure at home. Older individuals—particularly the very elderly—may have visual and hearing impairments and lack the dexterity necessary to use a sphygmomanometer/stethoscope combination; spouses, friends, or nurses can then be very helpful. We usually suggest that patients use an electronic sphygmomanometer that simply requires the cuff to be placed around the arm in the usual way (see Question 3); with the press of a button, the cuff automatically inflates and deflates, giving the systolic and diastolic pressures as well as the heart rate. The top-of-the-line Omron (HEM-704C) and Sunbeam (7650) electronic sphygmomanometers have been found to be highly accurate; nevertheless, their accuracy should be periodically validated by comparing their blood pressure determinations with those obtained with a mercury manometer. An extra-large cuff should be used for obese patients or individuals with large and muscular arms. The physician should help the patient select the proper-size cuff.

When measuring blood pressure at home, the patient should remember to remain seated, at rest, and relaxed in a quiet environment for at least five minutes before recording the data. Smoking, caffeine, and exercise should be avoided for one hour before taking the reading, and any stress should be avoided just prior to the measurement. Even talking has been reported to increase systolic and diastolic pressure. Another reason for using an electronic sphygmomanometer is that no physical activity is required to inflate the cuff, as even this small activity might increase blood pressure slightly. Because blood pressures are usually higher in the morning than in the afternoon or evening, it is helpful to record pressures periodically at different times of the day; the results may indicate the need for administering some medications more than once daily.

Home-based measurements of blood pressure have increased in popularity in recent years and are strongly recommended. They appear to be a very reliable guide for physicians treating hypertensive patients, and they seem to correlate well with target organ damage such as enlargement of the left ventricle of the heart (the main pumping chamber) and the occurrence of kidney damage. Note, however, that 24-hour blood pressure monitoring measurements are even more closely correlated with target organ damage involving the heart, kidney, eyes, and carotid arteries (the arteries that supply blood to the brain).

As previously mentioned, 24-hour ambulatory blood pressure monitoring can aid in identifying patients with suspected "white-coat hypertension" (see Question 14) and in assessing the effectiveness of antihypertensive treatment. In addition, it can prove especially valuable in linking symptoms of very low blood pressure to antihypertensive treatment and in correlating symptoms of an excessive excitation of the sympathetic nervous system or excessive hormones (adrenaline and noradrenaline) in the circulation with episodic hypertension accompanied by a rapid heart rate, profuse sweating, and headache (see Question 35). Likewise, 24-hour monitoring may supply important information about individuals thought to be suffering from sleep apnea. Nevertheless, this type of monitoring is very rarely needed in the management of hypertension.

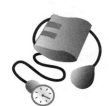

20. Which Blood Pressure Is More Important— Systolic or Diastolic?

It now appears that elevated systolic pressure is a greater risk factor for complications of hypertension than elevated diastolic pressure (see Question 2). For many years diastolic blood pressure was considered more important, probably because the blood vessels are subjected to this type of pressure most of the time (between heartbeats). Recently, however, observational studies have confirmed that systolic blood pressure is actually a better predictor of strokes, heart attacks, heart failure, kidney disease, and overall mortality. Data suggest that pulse pressure (the difference between the systolic and diastolic pressures—that is, systolic pressure minus diastolic pressure) may eventually turn out to be even more important than either systolic or diastolic blood pressure. For now, the evidence suggests that systolic pressure is more important than diastolic pressure in determining a person's risk of developing hypertension complications.

Elevated systolic pressure is a greater risk factor for complications of hypertension than elevated diastolic pressure.

Elevation of only systolic pressure (so-called isolated systolic hypertension) occurs quite frequently in older individuals and usually results from "hardening" (arteriosclerosis) of the large arteries. This physical change may be accompanied by significant arteriosclerosis in the arteries of the heart and brain, which increases the likelihood of stroke and heart attack. Elevated diastolic pressure is less accurate than systolic pressure as a predictor of complications of hypertension, especially in elderly patients.

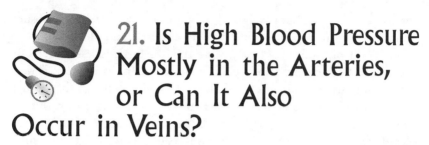

21. Is High Blood Pressure Mostly in the Arteries, or Can It Also Occur in Veins?

The high blood pressure discussed in this book is "arterial hypertension"— that is, high blood pressure in the arteries. Pressure in the veins, which is normally much lower than pressure in the arteries, is not affected in such hypertension, although it may sometimes be high due to heart failure or obstruction in the veins (not related to arterial hypertension). This fact undoubtedly explains why the damage from high blood pressure occurs in the arteries and not in the veins.

"Arterial hypertension" involves high blood pressure in the arteries.

To refresh your memory, arteries carry blood from the heart to the organs and tissues, which are in turn fed by tiny, microscopic vessels called capillaries. The arterioles (the smallest arteries) are microscopic, muscular extensions of the arteries found before the arterial system breaks up into capillaries. Most authorities believe that high blood pressure occurs because of greater than normal constriction of the arterioles, which produces resistance to the flow of blood in the arteries (see Questions 1, 6, 13). The veins are thin-walled vessels that return blood from the tissues to the heart and lungs and that are not affected by hypertension.

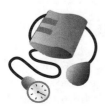

22. Is It Normal for Blood Pressure to Increase with Age?

It is probably not normal for blood pressure to increase with age. In the United States and other industrialized societies such as Western Europe, blood pressure *does* increase with age, but this occurrence does not necessarily make it "normal." In lesser acculturated (more primitive) societies, such as Indian tribes in the Amazon jungles of Brazil and inhabitants of remote regions of the South Pacific, blood pressure stays low (by Western standards) throughout life. **The Western lifestyle may be the culprit in the tendency of blood pressure to increase with age.** "Low blood pressure" populations are characterized by diets low in saturated fat and salt, vigorous exercise, lean body weight throughout life, and lack of exposure to industrialization, which to some implies a more tranquil lifestyle.

The blood pressure of infants at the time of birth is less than 100/60 mm Hg in both civilized and primitive societies. In primitive societies, blood pressure usually remains at that level throughout life. In the United States, however, it is considered "normal" for blood pressure to rise during the first 20 years of life. This measurement is not considered "high" until it exceeds 136/87 mm Hg for 17-year-old boys of average height; for girls, blood pressure is slightly less. Because of progressive "hardening" (arteriosclerosis) of the large arteries, systolic blood pressure tends to increase with age throughout life for both men and women in the United States. This "average" increase should not be considered normal—the progressive elevation of blood pressure accounts for the high morbidity and mortality rate from cardiovascular disease in elderly Americans. The old adage that systolic blood pressure should be 100 plus your age is both unhealthy and untrue. The average diastolic blood pressure in the United States tends to increase until age 50–55, then begins to decline. This change indicates that high pulse pressures (the difference between systolic and diastolic pressures) are unhealthy and result from aging.

The old adage that systolic blood pressure should be 100 plus your age is both unhealthy and untrue.

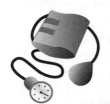

23. Can Stress Cause Hypertension and How Can You Reduce Stress?

Although some people think that hypertension means that they are "hyper-tense," in reality hypertension simply means "high blood pressure." Nevertheless, emotional tension or stress can result from unpleasant physical or mental stimuli and is usually associated with a transitory increase in heart and respiratory rates and blood pressure (see Question 9). This transformation is a normal response that we all experience, and the blood pressure returns to its original level after removal of stress. The notion that stress is a *major* cause of *permanent* hypertension is incorrect. Stressful events occur in the lives of all humans, and the release of hormones by the adrenal glands can be valuable in increasing alertness, fueling the competitive drive, and enhancing athletic performance.

> *The notion that stress is a major cause of permanent hypertension is incorrect.*

The response to various types of stress differs from person to person. For example, the anxiety and emotional stress of having one's blood pressure taken by a doctor cause 20% of patients to experience "white-coat hypertension" (see Question 14). Although stress can trigger a "fight or flight" reaction occasioned by anticipation of physical conflict, the response can vary significantly among individuals. The elevated blood pressure caused by the discomfort of placing one's hand in ice water for one minute (the "cold pressor test") also results in varying degrees of blood pressure elevation in different subjects (see Question 36). While the response to stress is usually greater in men than women, the stress response to a crying baby has been reported to be greater in women than it is in men.

One investigator reported some fascinating observations of blood pressure change, which he recorded frequently with an electronic device during a 24-hour period. Even talking on the telephone was found to raise pressure by 5 mm Hg; in contrast, relaxing or watching TV caused the pressure to drop. In this study, the highest blood pressure measurements were recorded at work or during commuting. In the evening after work, unmarried women usually experienced a decrease in pressure; the blood pressure in married women with children did not decrease during this time, however. Men's blood pressures usually declined in the evening regardless of whether they had children. It was suggested that women with young children have two causes of stress: (1) their jobs during the day and (2) their family responsibilities during the evening. Nevertheless, no evidence indicates that women who have full-time jobs during the day and a family to care for in the evening are more likely to develop hypertension.

Although it might seem reasonable to believe that repeated, pronounced elevations of blood pressure can damage blood vessels and increase the occurrence of stroke and heart attack, no strong evidence confirms this occurrence in persons with normal blood pressure. Furthermore, no evidence indicates that individuals with type A personalities (highly competitive, ambitious, aggressive, impatient, perfectionist) are more prone to hypertension than any other persons (see Question 10). Some studies have found that men with stressful jobs over which they have no control are more prone to eventually develop hypertension and heart attacks, especially if they are blue-collar workers with limited education. Particularly noteworthy is the finding that air traffic controllers, who are exposed to considerable amounts of psychological stress, develop hypertension at a rate 5.6 times greater than do pilots who share similar physical characteristics. In addition, men who are continually striving to improve their lifestyle status and live beyond their financial means are more likely to develop hypertension than men who remain content with the status quo. In contrast, people living in protected and secluded societies (for example, nuns) have been found to maintain relatively low blood pressures throughout life. In individuals with hypertension, stress may further aggravate hypertension and increase the risk of arterial damage, stroke, and heart attack.

Clearly, some people handle stress much better than others. The response to stress depends on the amount and type of stress and its duration. Under certain circumstances, prolonged psychological stress may contribute to the development of sustained hypertension in some individuals.

As mentioned earlier, a sudden and very stressful event may cause severe anxiety accompanied by a pronounced increase in blood pressure and heart rate with excessive perspiration. This response ends when the stress is removed. Occasionally, however, a sudden rise in blood pressure and heart rate may cause an irregular heart beat, pain or a pressure sensation in the chest (angina), and even a heart attack in persons with impaired circulation in the heart.

In contrast, chronic stress may result in fatigue, irritability, headache, inability to concentrate, insomnia, depression, discouragement, frequent complaints, and unhappiness. Work performance may be disrupted, and family life can suffer disastrous consequences. Chronic stress may make an individual feel trapped with no way out, no escape hatch. Furthermore, it may suppress the immune system and make an individual more susceptible to infections and malignant tumors. Nevertheless, chronic stress does not cause persistent hypertension.

The management of stress, which recurs on a daily basis, can be difficult. Certain basic steps may prove very helpful in this regard:

1. **Adequate sleep—at least seven hours each night—is important.** Over-the-counter sleep medication (usually a pain reliever plus an antihistamine, such as Tylenol PM) may be very helpful. Only rarely are prescription drugs indicated to induce sleep, because they can be habit-forming.

2. **Eating a healthy and moderate-size meal at least two hours before retiring and consuming no more than one or two alcoholic drinks**

with the evening meal is recommended. Consumption of a large meal and excess alcohol may interfere with sleep.

3. **Getting adequate aerobic exercise (30 minutes per day, 5 days per week) on a regular basis is critical.** Exercise is not only good for your physical condition, but can also have a remarkably beneficial effect on emotional tension. Physical conditioning and maintaining appropriate weight can improve your appearance, make you feel good about yourself, and relieve some of the stress that may result from being inactive and overweight.

Of some interest are reports that stress relief and lower blood pressure may be benefits for some individuals who develop a strong attachment and warm affection for pets (for example, dogs and cats).

Avoiding conflict, maintaining a positive attitude, scheduling work to avoid being rushed at the last minute, avoiding inessential duties, getting adequate vacation time, pursuing muscle relaxation techniques (for example, closing your eyes while you are in a seated or recumbent position and then in gradual sequence concentrating on relaxing muscles in the feet, then legs, hips, abdomen, hands, arms, neck, and face), meditating, and performing biofeedback may prove beneficial in stress management. Unfortunately, these tactics are ineffective in the treatment of chronic hypertension. If stress continues and becomes intolerable, then drugs that reduce tension without significantly impairing performance, and psychiatric consultation may be appropriate.

> *Avoiding conflict, maintaining a positive attitude, scheduling work to avoid being rushed at the last minute, avoiding inessential duties, getting adequate vacation time, and pursuing muscle relaxation techniques, meditation, and biofeedback may prove beneficial in stress management.*

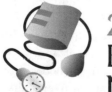

24. Does Alcohol Increase Blood Pressure? How Much Can I Drink If I Have Hypertension?

Perhaps 7% to 10% of all cases of hypertension in the United States are caused by excess alcohol consumption. This percentage is considerably higher in communities and countries where many individuals drink alcohol in excessive amounts.

Men with hypertension who consume alcohol should limit their intake to no more than two ounces of 80- to 100-proof spirits, two cans of beer, or two glasses of wine each day (equivalent to one ounce of ethanol). Women or small men should limit their intake to half this amount. Restricting alcohol consumption is especially important for hypertensive women, because they have less of the enzyme alcohol dehydrogenase in their stomach than men; this enzyme is important in metabolizing alcohol. The moderate amount of alcohol consumption recommended here rarely causes an elevation of blood pressure and even appears to decrease the occurrence of heart attacks when compared to teetotalers. If you have hypertension and find that even this moderate consumption of alcohol increases your blood pressure, then you should not drink alcohol.

Men with hypertension who consume alcohol should limit their intake to no more than two ounces of 80- to 100-proof spirits, two cans of beer, or two glasses of wine each day. Women or small men should limit their intake to half this amount.

Note that alcohol consumption provides a significant number of calories (one bottle of beer contains 100 to 150 calories, and one glass of wine contains approximately 125 calories) without any nutritional benefit. This point is worth remembering if you are hypertensive and trying to lose weight. Modest alcohol intake may slightly elevate the level of "good" cholesterol [high-density (HDL) lipoprotein], which protects arteries from accumulating cholesterol deposits. Nevertheless, alcohol consumption should certainly be limited in hypertensive individuals.

Evidence gathered in France has suggested that consumption of red wine may protect individuals from heart attacks. Although the precise explanation for this effect remains to be elucidated, a chemical in the wine, which decreases the tendency of blood to clot, may play a role. Before endorsing the consumption of red or white wine, one should take heed of the fact that excess consumption of wine in France accounts for the highest incidence of cirrhosis (liver disease) in the world.

The reason why excess alcohol elevates blood pressure is uncertain. The lower blood pressure associated with a reduction of excess alcohol consumption can be impressive—systolic and diastolic pressure may decrease as much as 13 mm Hg and 7 mm Hg, respectively. If a heavy drinker wishes to curtail his or her alcohol consumption, this reduction should occur gradually. Abrupt cessation of alcohol intake can stimulate the sympathetic nervous system by liberating hormones (adrenaline and noradrenaline), which can then constrict arteries and sometimes cause severe hypertension. Heavy drinkers should consult a physician and develop a program for cessation of drinking so as to minimize or prevent symptoms of alcohol withdrawal such as anxiety, shakiness, insomnia, increased pulse, temperature, and respiration, upset stomach, and sometimes confusion and hallucinations.

Finally, it should be noted that alcohol consumption may enhance the effects of some antihypertensive medications, leading to a decrease in blood pressure that may cause one to feel faint and unsteady. This interaction could be particularly hazardous while driving a car.

25. Does High Blood Pressure Occur in Children, and Should Children and Adolescents with Essential Hypertension Be Treated?

High blood pressure does indeed occur in children—and more frequently than we thought before pediatricians started measuring blood pressure in children on routine office visits. Remember that "normal" blood pressure for children is lower than it is for adults. For instance, at age 1 year, the upper limit of "normal" is 104/58 mm Hg for a girl of average height and 102/57 mm Hg for a boy of average height. By age 17, these upper limits of normal have increased to 129/84 mm Hg for a girl and 136/87 mm Hg for a boy. Pediatricians believe that blood pressure in children should be related to their height. Perhaps our willingness to accept a rise in blood pressure with age as "normal" explains why so much cardiovascular disease is found in industrialized nations.

Pediatricians would prefer to manage hypertension in children and adolescents with lifestyle modifications, if possible. If these measures fail, drugs are recommended with appropriate modification of doses depending on body weight.

Pediatricians would prefer to manage hypertension in children and adolescents with lifestyle modifications, if possible. Such a strategy would include weight reduction when the patient is obese, reduction of salt in the diet to no more than 6 grams (g) per day, and adequate aerobic exercise, unless some reason exists to avoid exercise. In short, hypertensive children and adolescents should avoid excess dietary fat and "fast food" to which most of them are addicted. Hypertension should not restrict children's participation in sports, unless the blood pressure is very high. After blood pressure has been successfully lowered, exercise can still prove very beneficial.

If these measures fail to modify the hypertension, drugs are recommended with appropriate modification of doses depending upon body weight. ACE inhibitors and angiotensin II receptor blockers should not be prescribed for pregnant or sexually active girls (see Question 66).

Finally, it is important to recognize that hypertension, particularly if severe, in children and adolescents is often due to secondary causes (see Question 38).

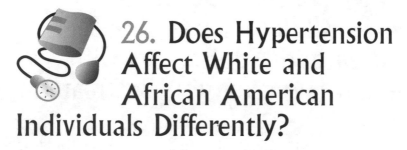

26. Does Hypertension Affect White and African American Individuals Differently?

African Americans of any age are more likely to have hypertension than their white counterparts. Not only does hypertension occur more frequently in the African American population, but it is also more severe. In addition, African American individuals are more likely to have complications earlier in the course of the disease. The mortality rate for stroke is 80% higher and the mortality rate for heart disease is 50% higher in African Americans than the corresponding rates in whites. Kidney complications with kidney failure are 325% more frequently observed in African Americans than in whites.

African Americans of any age are more likely to have hypertension than their white counterparts. Not only does hypertension occur more frequently in the African American population, but it is also more severe.

The explanation for the greater prevalence and severity of hypertension in African Americans than white individuals remains to be elucidated (see Question 34). However, approximately 60% of hypertensive persons are salt-sensitive—that is, their blood pressure becomes significantly elevated when they consume excess amounts of salt. Salt sensitivity may result from a genetic kidney abnormality, which causes retention of excess amounts of salt; this combination appears especially common in African Americans. Excess salt consumption by individuals who are salt-sensitive will, of course, aggravate hypertension and its severity.

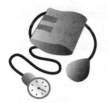

27. What Is Malignant Hypertension?

"Malignant hypertension"—the most severe form of hypertension—is rapidly progressive and leads quickly to target organ damage. Unless properly treated, it is fatal within five years for about 90% of its victims. Death usually comes from congestive heart failure, kidney failure, or brain hemorrhage.

It is not possible to diagnose malignant hypertension by measuring blood pressure, because many hypertensive patients who lack this condition will have blood pressures as high as those who do have it. Patients with malignant hypertension characteristically demonstrate tiny hemorrhages and exudates (white spots) in the retina at the back of the eyes. The optic nerve seen in the back of each eye may be swollen (papilledema). Fortunately, aggressive treatment can reverse malignant hypertension and prevent its complications. In fact, this type of hypertension is now quite rare, whereas 30 or 40 years ago (before the advent of effective drugs) it was much more common. **Malignant hypertension is not attributable to cancer or a malignancy, although the rapidly fatal outcomes are much worse than those associated with most malignancies.**

> *"Malignant hypertension"—the most severe form of hypertension—is rapidly progressive and leads quickly to target organ damage. Unless properly treated, it is fatal within five years for about 90% of its victims.*

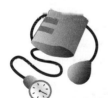

28. Why Is Essential Hypertension Called "The Silent Killer"? Is It a Disease?

In one sense, it is unfortunate that the most common type of high blood pressure—essential or primary hypertension—very rarely causes symptoms or signs that warn individuals about their elevated blood pressure. As a consequence, complications of hypertension, including hardening of the arteries, stroke, heart attack, heart and kidney failure, impaired vision, and death, may occur before the blood pressure elevation is recognized—hence the name "the silent killer." Many people believe that a red or flushed appearance of the face is always a sign of hypertension and that headache is a common symptom of an elevated blood pressure; these notions are actually misconceptions (see Question 9). Mild headaches may occasionally affect some hypertensives, but only very rarely will a person with fairly severe hypertension experience a rather severe headache; some headaches are experienced in the morning and often subside on arising. It should be emphasized that **it is impossible for individuals to know whether their blood pressure is elevated by the way they feel** (see Question 9).

Essential or primary hypertension very rarely causes symptoms or signs that warn individuals about their elevated blood pressure. As a consequence, complications of hypertension may occur before the blood pressure elevation is recognized— hence the name "the silent killer."

Essential hypertension accounts for the elevated blood pressure in approximately 95% of the 50 million Americans with hypertension. It is more correct to consider high blood pressure to be an abnormal condition of the regulation of the circulation rather than a specific disease, as the causes of this form of hypertension remain unknown. Although genetic and environmental factors (especially obesity and excess salt consumption) are often directly related to the development of hypertension, exactly how each factor promotes hypertension remains unclear (see Questions 6, 13, 33).

With secondary types of hypertension, a specific disease causes the elevated blood pressure (see Question 38). Symptoms, signs, and certain biochemical abnormalities are frequently present with this type of hypertension, which can permit a physician to make a diagnosis at a relatively early stage of the disease.

Because essential hypertension may remain silent for many years and lead to serious complications, it is essential that everyone have their blood pressure checked at least every one to two years. This minimal investment of time may yield maximal dividends—protection and preservation of your health!

29. Can Thyroid Disease Be Causing My Hypertension, and What Are the Manifestations?

Both an overactive thyroid gland and an underactive thyroid gland can cause or aggravate hypertension. Nevertheless, abnormal thyroid function only sometimes causes hypertension.

Approximately 20% to 30% of patients with an overactive thyroid gland (hyperthyroidism) have hypertension. **This condition usually takes the form of mainly or only elevated systolic blood pressure; diastolic pressure is often decreased** (resulting in a widening of the pulse pressure—that is, the difference between the systolic and diastolic pressures). **Many patients with an overactive thyroid will, however, have some elevation of their diastolic pressure.** Their hypertension results from overproduction of the thyroid hormones, which stimulate the rate and pumping action of the heart.

In patients with hyperthyroidism, hypertension results from overproduction of the thyroid hormones, which stimulate the rate and pumping action of the heart, and usually cause characteristic manifestations.

Manifestations of hyperthyroidism are often readily apparent. The patient may have prominent eyes that give a scared or frightened appearance to the face, nervousness, trembling, emotional lability, heat intolerance, excess sweating, palpitations (heart consciousness), diarrhea, insomnia, weight loss despite increased appetite, decreased menstruation, fatigue, and a variety of less obvious manifestations. The entire thyroid gland is usually enlarged, but may have a discrete nodule or multiple nodules. In elderly patients, manifestations may be less obvious and perhaps include only cardiovascular symptoms such as angina (pain or pressure sensation in the chest) and irregularity of the heart rhythm. The diagnosis is easily established by blood tests, which reveal excess concentrations of the thyroid hormones. With appropriate treatment, the hypertension usually disappears or returns to its previous level.

A small percentage of the total hypertensive population has been reported to have an underactive thyroid gland, a condition known as hypothyroidism. **In individuals with hypothyroidism and hypertension, both systolic and diastolic pressures are elevated**, which appears to result from activation of the sympathetic nervous system and constriction of arterioles. These patients usually have a slow pulse and a decreased pumping action of the heart.

In patients with hypothyroidism, hypertension may result from activation of the sympathetic nervous system and constriction of arterioles. Deficiency of thyroid hormones may cause characteristic manifestations.

The manifestations of hypothyroidism may include fatigue, lethargy, a slowing of intellectual function and physical activity, cold intolerance, a deepening of the voice and sometimes hoarseness, and dry skin and hair with some hair loss. The thyroid gland is usually not enlarged, although a goiter (a very large thyroid) is sometimes readily evident. The diagnosis is easily confirmed by blood tests—the concentration of thyroid-stimulating hormone (TSH) is elevated in 95% of cases.

Replacement of the deficient thyroid hormone usually returns the blood pressure to its previous level.

Because of the characteristic manifestations of abnormal thyroid function and the availability of excellent blood tests for these conditions, it should not be difficult for the physician to determine whether thyroid malfunction is responsible for hypertension.

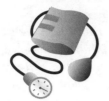

30. Can Hypertension Lead to Blindness?

Only rarely does hypertension lead to blindness. The eye is considered a "target organ" of hypertension, because this condition can damage the small blood vessels in the retina (the membrane at the back of the eye that senses images formed by the lens, which are transmitted to the brain). Nevertheless, hypertension rarely leads to various degrees of blindness (being "legally blind" implies very poor vision—unable to read, drive, or function without some help). When it does, the problem is usually temporary and eyesight improves with treatment of the hypertension.

An ophthalmoscope can be employed to look through the lens at small blood vessels in the retina, thereby enabling the physician to classify the severity of the hypertension even if eyesight is not affected. Evidence of hypertension as determined by the ophthalmoscope includes narrowing of retinal arterioles, hemorrhages, white patches (known as exudates) of various degrees, and swelling of the optic nerve, when the blood pressure remains very high for a prolonged period. All of these changes in the retina and optic nerve may impair vision.

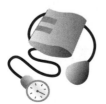

31. Can Hypertension Lead to Dialysis and How Does Dialysis Work?

Hypertension certainly can force the patient into dialysis. The kidneys are one of the "target organs" of hypertension. Untreated hypertension can lead to kidney failure with uremia (accumulation of waste products and chemicals in the blood), which requires dialysis or transplantation. Next to diabetes, the most frequent cause for patients to undergo dialysis or a kidney transplant is hypertension. The effects of dialysis on a person's lifestyle are devastating, and the yearly costs of dialysis may run as high as $100,000. The good news is that effective treatment of high blood pressure will prevent this complication. Treatment, however, should begin before damage to the kidneys occurs. Once such damage is present, treatment may slow down the process, but it will not entirely prevent or reverse the problem.

Dialysis is a means of removing waste products and undesirable chemicals from the blood of patients with acute or chronic kidney failure; chronic kidney failure is also known as end-stage renal (kidney) disease (ESRD). In hemodialysis, blood flows for about four hours from an artery through an artificial kidney and then back into a vein of the patient. The waste products and undesirable chemicals pass from the blood through a cellophane membrane into the dialyzing fluid, which is continually being discarded and replaced by a constant flow of fresh fluid. The "cleaned" blood returned to the body contains a much more normal composition than the blood before dialysis. Unfortunately, some patients may require dialysis several times each week.

> *Dialysis is a means of removing waste products and undesirable chemicals from the blood of patients with acute or chronic kidney failure.*

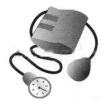

32. Can Hypertension Cause Alzheimer's Disease or Dementia?

No evidence indicates that hypertension causes Alzheimer's disease. Patients who have never had hypertension can develop Alzheimer's disease, and treatment of hypertension does not seem to improve the condition. Multiple small strokes, however, sometimes result in a condition similar to Alzheimer's that is marked by progressive dementia (memory loss), called "multi-infarct dementia." This type of dementia is related to hypertension because hypertension is a risk factor for strokes. Unfortunately, although treatment of high blood pressure may prevent strokes, it does not improve multi-infarct dementia once it has occurred.

33. Is Hypertension Ever Familial and Is There an Explanation for This Relationship?

There is a strong familial link in essential or primary hypertension, which accounts for 95% of all hypertension cases, the cause of which is not known. If one parent has essential hypertension, approximately 25% of his or her children will develop hypertension; if both parents have hypertension, the percentage of their children developing hypertension increases to 75% (see Questions 6, 13). The precise genetic defects that may explain this familial tendency to develop hypertension remain unclear, but it appears that multiple genes are involved and interact with one another and environmental factors. In addition, several hormonal systems and the sympathetic nervous system may play major roles in the development of hypertension.

There is a strong familial link in essential or primary hypertension, which accounts for 95% of all hypertension cases.

Notably, perhaps 50% to 60% of individuals with essential hypertension are salt-sensitive—that is, their blood pressure becomes elevated when they consume excess amounts of salt. Some evidence indicates that the kidneys in salt-sensitive animals retain more salt than the same organs in animals that are not salt-sensitive. It seems likely that a similar condition may exist in salt-sensitive humans. It is noteworthy that the prevalence of hypertension is greater in African Americans and that black individuals are more likely to be salt-sensitive than whites; furthermore, African Americans usually develop hypertension at a younger age than whites, and their hypertension is more severe and accompanied by more serious complications of cardiovascular disease than hypertension in whites. Although these differences between African Americans and whites have genetic implications, the abnormalities remain undefined as yet.

A single gene abnormality is responsible for polycystic kidney disease, which frequently causes hypertension in family members and relatives. Some of these patients have high amounts of renin in the blood released from the cystic kidneys; the renin generates angiotensin II, which can cause hypertension.

In addition, a number of very rare inherited conditions (accounting for about 0.2% of all hypertensives) cause hypertension because of a single gene defect:

- In *Liddle's syndrome*, a defect in the kidney tubules causes too much retention of salt and water.
- In *glucocorticoid remedial aldosteronism (GRA)*, the hypertension results from too much aldosterone hormone being produced by the adrenal glands, leading to excess retention of salt and water.
- In *congenital adrenal hyperplasia* (an enlargement of the adrenal glands), the hypertension results from an enzyme defect that leads to the production of a steroid, which causes retention of excess salt and water.

In these rare conditions, expansion of the blood volume results from salt and water retention and thereby increases the pumping action of the heart, which causes hypertension (see Question 38).

Another rare form of familial hypertension results from tumors of the adrenal glands that secrete adrenaline and noradrenaline, which can increase the pumping action of the heart and cause constriction of arterioles, thereby raising blood pressure. These rare familial tumors, which occur with other endocrine tumors and abnormalities, are known as multiple endocrine neoplasia (MEN) syndromes. A genetic abnormality has been detected in most patients with these tumors, and they can occur in many family members and their relatives (see Question 35).

Finally, **preeclampsia has a hereditary tendency.** This condition has been reported in 25% of daughters and granddaughters of patients who have experienced preeclampsia. As yet, the explanation for preeclampsia's development and familial occurrence remains unknown.

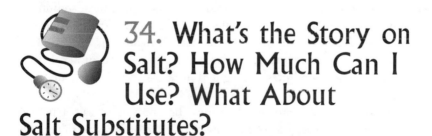

34. What's the Story on Salt? How Much Can I Use? What About Salt Substitutes?

Salt (sodium chloride) plays a role in causing high blood pressure in 50% to 60% of all people with hypertension. For example, adequate dietary salt restriction and increased salt elimination caused by diuretics (taking "water pills") can significantly lower blood pressure in some people with hypertension. In addition, a strong relationship has been proved to exist between the amount of salt eaten and hypertension. Finally, in certain experimental

Salt plays a role in causing high blood pressure in 50% to 60% of all people with hypertension.

animal models, including apes, unequivocal evidence shows that excess salt consumption causes hypertension.

Table salt is composed of 40% sodium and 60% chloride. Although it was previously thought that sodium alone was responsible for elevating blood pressure, researchers now believe that the combination of both sodium *and* chloride is required to produce hypertension in experimental animals and humans; sodium combined with substances other than chloride will not produce hypertension (see Question 13).

In the hypertensive population, roughly 75% of African Americans and 50% of white persons are salt-sensitive. Salt sensitivity is also particularly common in obese individuals, diabetics, and persons older than 65 years. The only way to find out whether you are sensitive to salt is to see whether going from a low-salt to a high-salt diet significantly increases your blood pressure, or vice versa. Excess salt consumption appears to decrease blood flow and salt excretion by the kidneys of salt-sensitive persons, whereas the kidneys of normal individuals increase their blood flow and excretion of salt under the same circumstances. Excess amounts of salt cause constriction of arterioles in salt-sensitive individuals, thereby increasing blood pressure; the reason for this arterial constriction remains unknown.

Although the greater occurrence and greater severity of hypertension in African Americans than in whites remains unexplained, it has been suggested that the kidneys of African Americans retain more salt than whites (see Question 26). Some African Americans may consume less potassium than whites, which may explain why they have more severe hypertension than whites; potassium appears to oppose the accumulation of sodium in the body and can dilate arteries and decrease blood pressure. In addition, a deficiency of calcium or magnesium may contribute to elevation of blood pressure. The exact interactions among sodium, potassium, calcium, and magnesium in blood pressure regulation remain to be elucidated (see Question 98).

Americans consume roughly 20 times the amount of salt a person requires for normal body function. More than 70% of ingested salt comes from processed food (that is, food prepared by companies for public consumption); one-sixth comes from natural, unprocessed food; and one-sixth is added in the household. Persons with hypertension should read the labels on processed foods to become familiar with the amounts of salt they are consuming.

Controversy continues to swirl over the question of whether the United States should implement a national policy to reduce salt consumption in the general population. Currently, the National High Blood Pressure Education Program (a coalition of about 45 national professional and federal agencies, of which the National Hypertension Association is a member) and the American Heart Association recommend a daily dietary intake of no more than 6 grams (g) of salt (sodium chloride); this is equivalent to 2400 mg of sodium. The average American now consumes about twice this amount. Reduction of salt intake to this level appears to be both safe and achievable, and it might reduce the number of people developing hypertension each year by 20% and decrease the yearly mortality rate from stroke and heart attack by 39% and 30%, respectively. Reducing dietary sodium may enhance the effectiveness of certain antihypertensive drugs and may eliminate the need of medication in some hypertensives.

The National High Blood Pressure Education Program and the American Heart Association recommend a daily dietary intake of no more than 6g of salt.

Limitation of salt intake should be combined with other healthful lifestyle changes, if indicated, such as weight reduction, smoking cessation, limited consumption of alcohol, adequate exercise, and consumption of a diet low in saturated fats and cholesterol (which is mainly found in animal tissues and dairy products) and high in fiber, fruits, and vegetables. Fresh foods have very little salt, and the addition of pepper, spices, herbs, lemon, onion, garlic, vinegar, table wine, horseradish, unsalted mustard, catsup (no added salt), and Worcestershire sauce (with low sodium) can add flavor to your food and help you kick the salt habit.

Some common foods high in sodium are listed in Table 3. Beware of particularly high sources of sodium! These items include tomato juice, cocoa mix, canned soups and vegetables, bologna and smoked meats, bacon, frankfurters, ham, tuna in oil, anchovies, sardines, pancake mix, salted potato chips, pretzels, popcorn, nuts, English muffins, bread, waffles, butter, cheese, bouillon, catsup, dill pickles, sauerkraut, and baking powder/soda.

Salt substitutes and "lite salt" should not be used without the recommendation of a physician. Many substitutes contain potassium chloride, which may be hazardous to some individuals—particularly those with impaired kidney function or those taking certain antihypertensive drugs that cause potassium retention. Evidence indicates that potassium may produce a beneficial effect by replacing sodium in cells and eliminating sodium in the urine, thereby lowering blood pressure. We also caution against the use of salt tablets to counteract salt and water loss, even with excess sweating in hot weather, unless recommended by a physician. For individuals who are particularly fond of salt, it is comforting to note that limiting salt in your diet will eventually decrease your desire for this compound and may actually make food taste better without it. So, "bon appetit"!

Table 3. *Examples of Common Foods with High Sodium Levels*

Food	Amount	Sodium (mg)
Bouillon, canned	1 cup	782
Canned juice, tomato	½ cup	438
Canned meat	1 oz	394
Canned soup, chicken noodle	1 cup	849
Canned soup, lentil with ham	1 cup	1319
Canned spaghetti and meatballs	1 cup	940
Cheeses:	1 oz	
Cream	1 oz	84
Swiss	1 oz	73
American, processed	1 oz	405
Low-sodium cheddar or colby	1 oz	6
Frankfurter, beef	1 serving	461
Canned olives	3	120
Pickles, dill	1 spear	384
Pizza, cheese	1 slice	336
Pot pie, beef	1 serving	736
Pot pie, turkey	1 serving	1390
Salad dressing, Thousand Island	1 tbsp	109
Italian sausage	1 link	665
Soy sauce	1 tbsp	1005
Frozen dinner, fried chicken with mashed potatoes and corn	1 serving	1500
Frozen dinner, meatloaf with mashed potatoes and carrots	1 serving	1943

Source: U.S. Department of Agriculture, Agricultural Research Service. USDA nutrient database for standard reference, release 13. 1999. Nutrient Data Laboratory home page, http://www.nal.usda.gov/fnic/foodcomp.

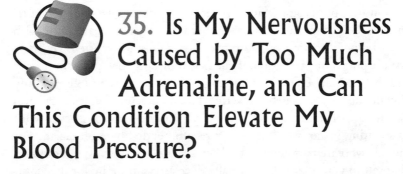

35. Is My Nervousness Caused by Too Much Adrenaline, and Can This Condition Elevate My Blood Pressure?

If you feel nervous, anxious, tense, apprehensive, or fearful, and you experience a rapid and pounding heart beat with elevated blood pressure and sometimes with sweating, it is reasonable to wonder whether too much of the adrenaline hormone is present in your circulation. Although an overactive sympathetic nervous system may partly explain your emotional disturbance, it is not ordinarily accompanied by any increase in the circulation of either adrenaline (released from the adrenal gland) or noradrenaline (released from sympathetic nerves). On the other hand, when strenuous exercise or emotional anxiety activates the "fight or flight" response, a modest increase of these hormones in the blood can occur and may be associated with transitory hypertension and a rapid heart rate.

An overactive sympathetic nervous system is not ordinarily accompanied by any increase in the circulation of either adrenaline or noradrenaline. On the other hand, a modest increase of these hormones in the blood can occur with the "fight or flight" response and be associated with transitory hypertension and a rapid heart rate.

Nevertheless, a rare but treacherous and potentially lethal tumor known as a pheochromocytoma (fe-o-kro' mo-si-to' mah) can cause enormous increases of adrenaline and noradrenaline in the blood. This condition produces either sustained or periodic elevations of blood pressure as well as a rapid heart rate (see Questions 33, 36, 38). Approximately 90% of such tumors arise in the adrenal glands, which are located on the top of each kidney. In some patients, they arise elsewhere in the abdomen (including the urinary bladder) and on rare occasions in the chest or neck. Roughly 10% of pheochromocytomas are familial (occurring in the same family or in relatives), and these cases may be associated with cancers of the thyroid gland and tumors of the parathyroid glands. Occasionally, patients with this familial disease will have nodules on the lips and tongue and other manifestations. Although pheochromocytoma is a rare cause of hypertension—occurring perhaps only once in every 2000 patients with both systolic and diastolic hypertension—it requires special vigilance by the physician to detect this "needle in the haystack" so that it can be promptly removed.

Most commonly, persons with a pheochromocytoma complain of headaches, sweating for no apparent reason, and a rapid heart rate with palpitations (the feeling that the heart is pounding and stronger than usual). There is often extreme pallor of the face (rarely flushing), sometimes a tremor of the hands, and occasionally marked apprehension and fear of impending death. Abdominal and chest pain; weight loss; visual disturbances; numbness, tingling, and pain in the extremities; and constipation or diarrhea may be experienced by some patients. Rarely, fever may occur and suggest an infection.

Most symptoms and signs occur repeatedly in a dramatic and explosive manner without any warning and may be experienced several times each day or only every few months. Because of the explosive nature of these attacks, pheochromocytoma has been described as a pharmacological bomb or a volcano that erupts periodically. These periodic attacks usually last about 15 minutes but may sometimes persist for hours, leaving the individual exhausted after the attack subsides. The blood pressure is often markedly elevated during these events but may remain normal between them, if the tumors release adrenaline and noradrenaline only periodically. If these hormones are released into the blood continuously, then the blood pressure may remain persistently elevated. In such cases, symptoms and signs may be experienced chronically but less severely than when attacks occur periodically. Attacks may sometimes be precipitated by pressure in the area of the tumor, change in posture, exercise, anxiety, ingestion of certain foods or alcoholic beverages, consumption of fruit juice, hyperventilation, straining, smoking, sexual intercourse, administration of certain drugs, operative manipulation, and child birth. If the tumor is located in the urinary bladder, attacks may be precipitated by bladder distention or urination.

The large number and great variety of manifestations associated with excess adrenaline and noradrenaline in the circulation have been referred to as kaleidoscopic. Pheochromocytoma has been called the "Great Mimic" or "Great Masquerader," because its symptoms and signs may simulate those linked to many other medical conditions—panic attacks, overactive thyroid gland, overactive heart and circulation, essential hypertension with and without widely fluctuating blood pressure, menopause, migraine and cluster headaches, low blood sugar, toxemia of pregnancy, inadequate circulation to the heart due to coronary artery disease, mitral valve prolapse (an incompetent valve in the heart), spinal cord injury, certain disturbances of brain function, infections, drugs that cause sudden hypertension, and a number of less common conditions. On rare occasions, adrenaline and noradrenaline will damage the heart muscle and cause heart failure. These hormones engender some biochemical changes—for example, blood sugar may be significantly elevated and suggest a diagnosis of diabetes.

Because approximately 95% of patients with pheochromocytoma are symptomatic, a detailed history and physical examination can prove valuable in determining which patients with sustained or intermittent hypertension should be screened for these tumors. All symptomatic patients with sustained or labile hypertension should be screened by measuring the levels of these hormones (or their metabolites), as pheochromocytomas secrete these substances into either the urine or blood. Once the diagnosis has been established, the tumor must be located by radiological techniques (such as a CAT scan), magnetic resonance imaging (MRI), or use of a radiolabeled substance that seeks out the tumor. Familial pheochromocytoma is often more difficult to diagnose than the nonfamilial version of the disease, because the former tumors tend to cause few (if any) symptoms and may not cause an elevated blood pressure. In such cases, blood and urine concentrations of adrenaline and noradrenaline and their metabolites, as well as the results of imaging, radiologic, and genetic studies, can help make the diagnosis and establish pheochromocytoma in other family members. Tumors of the eyes, brain, spinal cord, and skin are sometimes genetically related to pheochromocytomas.

The importance of recognizing this rare cause of hypertension cannot be overemphasized. With skillful management, the tumor can be removed successfully in 90% of cases; if it goes unrecognized or the diagnosis is made incorrectly, it will almost certainly prove fatal or cause catastrophic complications. Pheochromocytoma is always a challenge to the acumen of the physician. The dictum for the physician is, "Think of it, confirm it, locate it, and remove it!" If you have any of the manifestations caused by pheochromocytoma, you should mention them to your physician. Only very rarely are patients with signs and symptoms of excess adrenaline and noradrenaline harboring a pheochromocytoma; in such cases, however, the proper diagnosis must be either confirmed or excluded so as to avoid the serious, and perhaps lethal consequences of an unrecognized tumor.

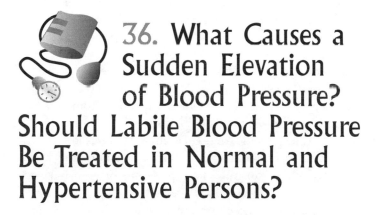

36. What Causes a Sudden Elevation of Blood Pressure? Should Labile Blood Pressure Be Treated in Normal and Hypertensive Persons?

Blood pressure fluctuates remarkably in both normal individuals and those with hypertension. Furthermore, this lability of blood pressure varies among different persons and is influenced by many factors.

Stimulation of the sympathetic nervous system can cause constriction of blood vessels and an increased pumping action of the heart, which in turn elevates blood pressure (see Question 13). This increase in sympathetic nervous system activity and blood pressure is greater in the morning and when a person first arises. Consequently, blood pressure is usually higher in the morning than in the evening, and it is lowest during sleep. During routine daily activities, however, the blood pressure can become rapidly elevated to a significant degree. For example, physical activity will increase blood pressure—with the effect being especially pronounced during strenuous aerobic exercise. Anaerobic exercise such as weightlifting may sometimes increase pressure to as high as 300 mm Hg!

In addition, the anxiety of having one's blood pressure taken by the doctor may cause a pronounced blood pressure elevation in about 20% of people who do not have hypertension (see Question 14). Experiencing pain or placing one's hand in ice water for one minute (the cold pressor test) can increase blood pressure dramatically in some individuals (see Question 23). Likewise, the fear and anger that may occur during a hostile encounter or the fright of a dangerous or threatening experience (for example, almost being struck by a car) can powerfully stimulate the sympathetic nervous system and produce a marked rise in blood pressure, accompanied by a rapid heart beat and a pounding in the chest. This reaction, due to activation of the sympathetic nerves and the release of adrenaline, was termed the "fight or flight" response by the late physiologist Walter Canon.

Some illicit drugs—especially cocaine, amphetamine, and some herbal remedies such as ephedra, which contains ephedrine—can cause marked transitory hypertension, which may rarely be lethal (see Question 71). A rare cause of marked elevations of blood pressure is a tumor which periodically releases hormones (adrenaline and noradrenaline) into the circulation (see Questions 35, 38). Usually this condition is associated with severe headaches, sweating, pallor, and pounding of the heart.

When blood pressure is monitored for 24 hours, the marked variability in normal persons is very obvious. Caffeine, nicotine from cigarette smoking, or an evening of excessive alcohol consumption can transiently elevate blood pressure. The periodic stress encountered in one's job or associated with family and social problems can also transiently raise blood pressure. In fact, mentally performing math problems or even having a conversation may transiently elevate blood pressure.

It is noteworthy, however, that blood pressure lability to the various stimuli mentioned previously is usually considerably greater in patients with untreated hypertension. This hyperlability of blood pressure is probably best explained by the fact that the arteries of hypertensive patients are already abnormally constricted and that any additional constriction caused by activation of the sympathetic nervous system results in an exaggerated blood pressure elevation. The arteries of hypertensive subjects appear to be especially responsive to the various stimuli that cause constriction of blood vessels.

In summary, a large array of physical and emotional factors may cause fluctuations of blood pressure throughout the day; some of these pressure elevations may be considerable even in normal individuals. No strong evidence exists to show that these transient elevations are a health risk. In contrast, the hyperlability seen in patients with untreated hypertension may damage blood vessels and increase the risk of heart attack, stroke, and heart and kidney failure. For this reason, hypertensive patients should be treated so as to minimize or eliminate excessive blood pressure fluctuations. If spontaneous marked elevations of blood pressure occur periodically, especially if accompanied by headaches, sweating, pounding of the heart, and pallor, the diagnosis of a tumor that secretes adrenaline-like hormones should be considered and the diagnosis confirmed or eliminated (see Question 35).

Transient elevations of blood pressure are not a health risk, but the hyperlability seen in patients with untreated hypertension may damage blood vessels and increase the risk of heart attack, stroke, and heart and kidney failure.

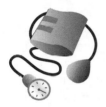

37. What Is Isolated Systolic Hypertension and Should It Be Treated?

The term "isolated systolic hypertension" (ISH) is used to describe the situation in which systolic blood pressure is elevated, but diastolic blood pressure is normal. For example, a blood pressure of 180/80 mm Hg would be considered ISH. This condition is especially common in elderly patients (usually older than 55 years) and is associated with increased risk of stroke, heart failure, and heart attacks. ISH in elderly patients is usually a reflection of widespread "hardening" of the large arteries (arteriosclerosis). ISH is uncommon in patients younger than 40 years of age. When it occurs in these individuals, it usually reflects an overactive heart that pumps increased amounts of blood; it is often a forerunner of systolic and diastolic hypertension later in life.

In isolated systolic hypertension, systolic blood pressure is elevated, but diastolic blood pressure is normal.

Persons with elevations of only their systolic blood pressure should always be treated. For many years, the decision to treat systolic blood pressure elevation was a source of concern and debate among physicians. We now know that we can reduce blood pressure in people with this type of hypertension, and that lowering the systolic blood pressure is beneficial and not harmful as once feared. In fact, the benefits of treating ISH are even greater and more immediately realized than the benefits of treating systolic and diastolic hypertension in younger patients. Studies have shown a remarkable 50% decrease in heart failure in ISH patients who received treatment as compared with those who received a sugar pill [placebo (see Question 74)]; the former group also saw significant reductions in heart attacks and strokes, and mortality was reduced significantly.

38. What Are the Causes of Secondary Hypertension and How Can You Identify Them?

Only some 5% of the 50 million hypertensive individuals in the United States have an identifiable cause of their elevated blood pressure, and hence have secondary hypertension. The 95% of patients have primary (essential) hypertension, in which the precise cause of the condition remains unknown. The good news is that secondary hypertension can sometimes be cured with surgery or successfully treated with medication, and primary hypertension can be controlled with medication.

The following findings suggest the presence of secondary hypertension: the sudden onset of hypertension in childhood or after the age of 50 years, especially if it is severe and accompanied by unusual symptoms, if it is resistant to treatment with medication, if certain abnormalities are found on physical examination, and if no family history of hypertension exists. A large number of conditions can cause secondary hypertension, some of which are listed in Table 4. It is beyond the scope of this answer to discuss all of the underlying causes of such hypertension and the means of diagnosing each condition, so only the most frequent causes of secondary hypertension will be mentioned here.

Kidney damage and impaired function account for most secondary forms of hypertension. Various types of nephritis (inflammation) or damage to kidney tissue (e.g. diabetic nephropathy) can usually be easily detected by increased amounts of protein and blood cells in the urine and sometimes retention of chemicals in the blood that are

Table 4. *Major Secondary Causes of Hypertension*

Kidney damage (nephropathy) and/or impaired function	a.	Diseases involving kidney tissue (not curable)
		Glomerulonephritis (acute or chronic inflammation)
		Diabetic nephropathy
		Polycystic kidney disease
		Lupus nephropathy
		Drug-induced nephropathy
		Injury-induced kidney damage
	b.	Narrowing of artery or arteries to kidneys (sometimes curable)
		Atherosclerosis
		Fibromuscular disease
	c.	Liddle's syndrome (treatable but not curable)
Endocrine	a.	Adrenal tumors or overactivity of adrenal glands
		Aldosteronoma or excess aldosterone secretion (curable or treatable)
		Familial enzyme abnormalities causing release of excess aldosterone (not curable)
		Pheochromocytoma (usually curable)
		Cushing's syndrome or disease (sometimes curable)
	b.	Overactive thyroid gland (curable)
		Underactive thyroid gland (treatable)
	c.	Oral contraceptives (curable)
	d.	Acromegaly—overactive pituitary gland (curable)
	e.	Overactive parathyroid glands (sometimes curable)
Drugs, drinks, and food	a.	Anabolic steroids and corticosteroids
	b.	Illicit drugs (cocaine, amphetamine, Ecstasy)
	c.	Alcohol (also alcohol withdrawal for alcoholics)
	d.	Cyclosporine
	e.	Erythropoietin
	f.	Caffeine
	g.	Nicotine
	h.	Appetite suppressants
	i.	Nonsteroidal anti-inflammatory drugs (NSAIDs)
	j.	Licorice and chewing tobacco
	k.	Monoamine oxidase (MAO) inhibitors
	l.	Phenylpropanolamine
	m.	Rebound hypertension with clonidine withdrawal

(Drugs, drinks, and food items a–m bracketed as: curable)

Table 4. *Continued*

Coarctation	Constriction in any part of aorta (curable)
Preeclampsia (toxemia of pregnancy) or eclampsia	Occurs in third trimester of pregnancy (curable)
Nervous system disorders or diseases	a. Increased pressure on the brain b. Brain tumors c. Convulsive seizures d. Quadriplegia from spinal cord injury sometimes curable e. Infections f. Lead or mercury poisoning
Sleep apnea	Not clear whether treatment cures hypertension

Note: The causes listed in this table account for only 5% of all people with hypertension. You should discuss these secondary causes of hypertension with your physician to obtain more detailed information regarding treatment and curability.

ordinarily eliminated by normal kidneys. Polycystic kidneys can usually be felt in the abdomen because of their significant enlargement; the presence of these enlarged kidneys with cysts is easily demonstrated by imaging studies (such as ultrasound or X rays of the kidneys). Because polycystic kidney disease is due to a genetic defect, it often affects other family members as well as the patient (see Question 33).

A narrowing (stenosis) of an artery to one or both kidneys can cause significant ischemia (impaired blood supply) of kidney tissue, thereby stimulating release of an enzyme (renin). Renin release generates angiotensin, which causes constriction of arterioles and thus raises blood pressure. Stenosis of an artery to the kidney is the most common cause of secondary hypertension that is curable, but accounts for less than 3% of the hypertensive population. The stenosis usually results from atherosclerosis accompanied by cholesterol plaque formation and partial obstruction of blood flow to the kidney. This obstruction usually occurs in the elderly. Obstruction of kidney arteries may also result from fibromuscular dysplasia, an overgrowth of smooth muscle cells in the wall of these arteries. This condition is most often seen in young women, especially those who smoke cigarettes.

The sudden onset of hypertension in the elderly or young women combined with the presence of a certain type of murmur (bruit) in the abdomen near the kidneys suggests stenosis of a kidney artery. The physician must then determine whether the stenosis is responsible for the hypertension. Certain imaging techniques can reveal a constriction of the artery, accompanied by a reduced blood flow, and a blood test can determine whether levels of renin are abnormally elevated and responsible for the hypertension.

Liddle's syndrome is a very rare genetic abnormality of the kidney that causes excess sodium retention, which in turn expands blood volume and causes hypertension. It can be identified through blood tests (see Question 33).

After kidney-related conditions, endocrine-related defects—particularly tumors of the adrenal gland—are the next most common cause of secondary hypertension. *Aldosteronomas* arise from the outer portion of the adrenal gland. They secrete excess amounts of aldosterone, a hormone that retains sodium, which in turn significantly expands blood volume and promotes increased pumping of the heart, constriction of arterioles, and hypertension. These types of tumors may be responsible for hypertension in less than 1% of all such patients. Tests identify this condition by detecting increased amounts of aldosterone in the blood and urine as well as low levels of potassium and renin in the blood. Patients may complain of weakness, headaches, and increased urination. Excess aldosterone may also result from overgrowth and overactivity of the cells that produce aldosterone in the adrenal gland. These conditions can usually be identified by a CAT or MRI scan of the adrenal glands. In addition, several rare, inherited abnormalities of enzymes in the adrenal gland can lead to excess production of aldosterone or deoxycorticosterone (a similar hormone); extra amounts of these hormones cause retention of sodium, expand blood volume, and produce hypertension (see Question 33).

Pheochromocytomas account for about 0.05% of all hypertension cases. Most such tumors (90%) arise in the inner portion of the adrenal gland, although in some patients they may arise elsewhere in the abdomen and the pelvis, including in the area where the aorta divides to supply blood to the legs and in the urinary bladder. Occasionally, pheochromocytomas occur in the back portion of the chest near the spine and in the region of the heart; rarely, they occur in the neck. These tumors usually secrete adrenaline and noradrenaline, both of which increase the pumping action of the heart, constrict most arterioles, and elevate blood pressure. In studies, 50% of these tumors were found to cause sustained hypertension whereas 45% caused only periodic hypertension—often with dramatic manifestations such as severe headache, palpitations (heart consciousness), excess sweating, pallor, and severe anxiety. A small percentage of pheochromocytomas do not cause hypertension. Approximately 10% are inherited, with the patient having immediate family members and other relatives who suffer from the same problem. Pheochromocytomas can be identified by blood or urine tests, which show elevated levels of adrenaline or noradrenaline or their breakdown products. These tumors can be located by a CAT or MRI scan or radioactive techniques (see Question 35).

Cushing's syndrome and Cushing's disease result when the adrenal glands secrete excessive amounts of a hormone, cortisol, into the blood. The syndrome is frequently caused by administration of steroids (for example, prednisone) as a treatment for various diseases. Cortisol often causes hypertension and produces a very characteristic body appearance that includes abdominal obesity, excess body hair, a round "moon" face, purple streaks on the abdomen, and a protuberance of fatty tissue in the back of the neck termed "buffalo hump." Cushing's syndrome is more frequently observed in women and is often accompanied by emotional disturbances, lack of menstrual periods, fatigue, and easy bruising. Blood tests, CAT or MRI scans of the adrenal glands, and an MRI scan of the pituitary gland can usually pinpoint whether this endocrine condition is due to an adrenal or pituitary abnormality.

An overactive thyroid gland (the result of increased thyroid hormones) usually elevates systolic blood pressure but lowers diastolic blood pressure; in some patients, diastolic pressure may also be elevated. An enlarged thyroid gland, prominent eyes, excessive and inappropriate sweating, heat intolerance, diarrhea, weight loss, nervousness, a tremor of the hands, and rapid heart beat frequently occur in individuals with hyperthyroidism. The increased heart rate and pumping action of the heart caused by the presence of excessive amounts of thyroid hormone in the circulation is mainly responsible for the elevated blood pressure. The diagnosis is easily established through thyroid function tests (see Question 29).

An underactive thyroid gland (the result of decreased thyroid hormone) is associated with a slowing of the heart rate and a decreased pumping action of the heart; the arterioles constrict so as to maintain adequate circulation to the tissues, which increases blood pressure (especially the diastolic pressure). A deficiency of thyroid hormone in children can result in short stature, coarse features, impaired mental development, and other problems; an enlarged thyroid gland (goiter) is usually present in such patients. In adults, the symptoms of hypothyroidism may be mistakenly attributed to aging or a disease involving the nervous system. Patients often complain of fatigue, lethargy, cold intolerance, constipation, weight gain, slowing of intellectual and muscle activity, loss of hair, dry skin, and a hoarse voice. The thyroid gland is usually not enlarged unless a goiter is present. Blood testing of thyroid activity will establish the diagnosis (see Question 29).

Oral contraceptives rarely cause hypertension today, given their lower concentrations of estrogen and progesterone. Nevertheless, if hypertension occurs as a result of the "pill," it may be severe. In most women who experience this problem, blood pressure will return to normal levels two or three months after discontinuing use of the pill. The reasons why hypertension develops are unclear, although sodium retention, blood volume expansion, and increased pumping action of the heart may play roles.

Acromegaly results from the presence of excess growth hormone. This condition is characterized by gigantism (tall stature) with enlarging hands, feet, and jaw and coarsening of the facial features. Visual defects may arise if a pituitary tumor (usually the cause of excess growth hormone production) places pressure on the nerves to the eyes. Hypertension occurs in about 50% of acromegalics and may be related to sodium retention, an expanded blood volume with increased pumping action of the heart, and constriction of arterioles. The diagnosis of acromegaly is made by observing the characteristic body changes and elevated blood levels of growth hormone. An MRI of the brain can usually identify a pituitary tumor.

Overactive parathyroid glands in the neck cause the release of excess amounts of parathyroid hormone and an increased concentration of calcium in the blood. Elevated calcium levels rarely account for hypertension. Usually patients have no symptoms, but excess urination and water drinking, along with constipation, kidney stones, peptic ulcer, and loss of calcium from the bones may occur. Diagnosis can be made by identifying increased parathyroid hormone and calcium concentrations in the blood.

Some drugs, drinks, and food may elevate blood pressure (see Table 4). Some of these substances cause hypertension by activating the sympathetic nervous system, which causes constriction of arterioles and hypertension. Others promote the retention of sodium with expansion of blood volume and increased pumping action of the heart, as well as increased constriction of arterioles.

Coarctation is an inherited, congenital constriction of the aorta, which usually occurs in the chest just beyond the blood vessels carrying blood to the arms. In this condition, blood pressure is elevated in the arms and upper portion of the body, but decreased in the portion of the body below the constriction. In general, the hypertension in the upper body occurs when the constriction obstructs the blood flow; sometimes, however, constriction of arterioles throughout the body may result from increased activity of the sympathetic nerves and elevated levels of angiotensin in the blood. Frequently a murmur may be heard near the coarctation, but the presence of elevated pressure in the arms and low pressure in the legs and the characteristic results of imaging studies establish the diagnosis (see Question 13).

Preeclampsia should be suspected if hypertension, a significant increase of protein (albumin) in the urine, and fluid retention (manifested by rapid excessive weight gain and swelling of the ankles) occurs after the twentieth week of pregnancy (see Question 58). The cause of preeclampsia (toxemia of pregnancy) remains unknown. The blood pressure of patients with this condition should be carefully controlled. Preeclampsia may occasionally be followed by *eclampsia*—a condition characterized by severe hypertension, and sometimes swelling of the brain, and convulsions. Eclampsia proves fatal in 18% of cases. Preeclampsia can be cured and eclampsia prevented by delivery of the fetus.

A number of nervous system disorders or diseases may activate the sympathetic nervous system and cause arteriolar constriction and hypertension. MRI studies of the brain may be helpful in demonstrating brain abnormalities. Heavy metal poisoning can be demonstrated by elevated levels of the metals in the blood.

Sleep apnea usually occurs in middle-aged adults (2% of women and 4% of men); hypertension affects more than 50% of these individuals (see Question 61). Most sleep apnea results from airway obstruction, which is most commonly found in individuals with upper body obesity. Loud snoring and episodes of gasping frequently occur in persons with sleep apnea, and daytime drowsiness is common. An overnight sleep study can identify sleep apnea.

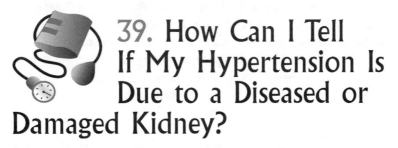

39. How Can I Tell If My Hypertension Is Due to a Diseased or Damaged Kidney?

Because the kidney is a target organ of hypertension and can also cause hypertension, it is sometimes difficult to tell whether kidney disease or damage caused the hypertension or resulted from it. If evidence of a kidney problem existed before the high blood pressure, then the kidney problem likely preceded the high blood pressure and, therefore, may have caused it. On the other hand, if no evidence of kidney disease existed before high blood pressure affected the patient for several years, then the kidney damage likely resulted from the hypertension.

Examination of blood and urine can help determine whether a kidney problem is present. Sometimes X rays employing contrast dyes—for example, intravenous pyelogram (which reveals the size of the kidneys and the structure that collects urine within the kidneys), kidney angiogram (which reveals the caliber of the arteries to the kidneys and identifies any obstruction to blood flow), or MRI angiogram (which may reveal abnormalities of the arteries to the kidneys without use of contrast material)—may be helpful. These imaging studies permit identification of damage to the kidneys and the arteries supplying them with blood.

In addition to being caused by a diseased or damaged kidney, hypertension can result from impaired blood supply to a kidney. This defect may promote the release of renin into the blood and the formation of angiotensin II. The latter causes constriction of arterioles, which in turn causes hypertension (see Question 38). Strokes, heart attacks, and heart failure are much more frequent complications of hypertension than kidney failure, and good control of high blood pressure can prevent or minimize kidney complications.

If evidence of a kidney problem existed before the high blood pressure, then the kidney problem likely preceded the high blood pressure and, therefore, may have caused it. If no evidence of kidney disease existed before high blood pressure affected the patient for several years, then the kidney damage likely resulted from the hypertension.

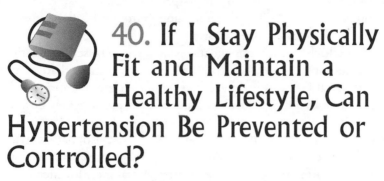

40. If I Stay Physically Fit and Maintain a Healthy Lifestyle, Can Hypertension Be Prevented or Controlled?

It would be wonderful if physical fitness could always prevent hypertension or reduce elevated blood pressure to a normal level. Unfortunately, it is frequently not effective in this regard. Maintaining physical fitness—through regular aerobic exercise, proper weight, avoidance of excess alcohol consumption, and abstinence from smoking—is certainly extremely desirable. Undoubtedly, adherence to such a program of physical fitness and consumption of a healthy diet are excellent means of sometimes preventing hypertension and reducing blood pressure. It is impossible to alter your genes, gender, age, and racial background, however. The genetic influence

Maintaining physical fitness may sometimes prevent hypertension or reduce elevated blood pressure to a normal level.

may be too powerful to enable physical fitness to prevent hypertension; furthermore, if blood pressure is constantly relatively high—for example, systolic and diastolic pressures greater than 165 and 110 mm Hg (millimeters of mercury), respectively—antihypertensive medication will almost certainly be required to normalize the pressure.

Weight loss appears to be the most effective means of lowering blood pressure without using antihypertensive drugs. Analysis of carefully controlled studies reveals that every kilogram (2.2 lb) of weight loss is accompanied by a fall in systolic and diastolic pressure of 1.6 and 1.3 mm Hg, respectively. In one study, a decrease of 23 lb resulted in a reduction of systolic and diastolic pressure by 11 and 8 mm Hg, respectively.

In our discussion of weight loss (see Question 48), we emphasize the importance of reducing caloric intake mainly by reducing fat to no more than 30% of total calories consumed. Low-fat diets matched with an abundance of fresh fruits and vegetables and little red meat will aid in lowering blood pressure. Increasing the expenditure of calories by undertaking regular aerobic exercise at least four or five times weekly is equally important for weight reduction. Finally, limiting salt consumption to approximately 6 grams (g) (1 teaspoonful), equivalent to 2400 milligrams of sodium, per day and restricting alcohol consumption to no more than one or two drinks of wine, beer, or spirits per day should be sufficient to prevent any hypertensive effect from alcohol or from salt, if the person happens to be salt-sensitive (see Question 34).

These lifestyle change recommendations are discussed elsewhere in this book (see Questions 24, 34, 46, 47, 49, 51, 88, 89). If these changes are made and physical fitness is maintained, a significant number of individuals with mild or even moderate elevations of blood pressure may be able to reduce their blood pressures to a normal range; furthermore, the development of hypertension may be prevented in perhaps 20% of persons who restrict their salt consumption to no more than 6 g per day. If lifestyle changes do not normalize blood pressure after several months, then antihypertensive drugs are indicated. Appropriate lifestyle changes will also lessen the amount of antihypertensive medication required to control blood pressure.

41. What Are Some of the Prescription and Over-the-Counter Drugs That Can Elevate Blood Pressure? What About Cold Medications?

It is important for patients with hypertension and even individuals without this condition to recognize that some over-the-counter (OTC) drugs may cause hypertension; furthermore, certain prescription drugs and some illicit drugs can also elevate blood pressure. For this reason, it is important to ask your doctor about any drug effects or interactions that could affect your pressure or prove harmful.

Drugs that can elevate blood pressure include some steroid or sex hormones, anesthetics, narcotics, illicit drugs, antidepressants, cyclosporine, erythropoietin, alcohol, disulfiram, appetite suppressants, phenylpropanolamine, nicotine, caffeine, licorice, nasal decongestants, salt-containing antacids, and nonsteroidal anti-inflammatory drugs.

Drugs that can elevate blood pressure include some steroid hormones, sex hormones, certain anesthetics, narcotics, illicit drugs, antidepressants, cyclosporine (a drug used to suppress the immune system), erythropoietin (used to correct anemias), alcohol, disulfiram (used in the treatment of alcoholics), appetite suppressants, phenylpropanolamine in diet pills, nicotine, caffeine, natural licorice or licorice added to chewing tobacco, nasal decongestants, antacids that contain lots of salt (sodium chloride), and nonsteroidal anti-inflammatory drugs (NSAIDs). Most of these drugs cause hypertension in one or more of three ways:

- By increasing retention of salt and water by the kidneys, which causes expansion of the blood volume and increases the pumping action of the heart
- By increasing the activity of the sympathetic nervous system, which leads to acceleration of the heart rate and constriction of arterioles
- By causing an accumulation of noradrenaline (a neurohormone) at sympathetic nerve endings, which then causes constriction of arterioles

All of these drug effects can, therefore, cause hypertension.

Many cold medications, "sinus medications," and decongestants contain ephedrine, pseudoephedrine, phenylephrine, or phenylpropanolamine; these ingredients can constrict the arteries and arterioles in the membranes lining the nasal cavity, thereby decreasing secretions of mucus and relieving the symptoms of nasal congestion. Although inhaling massive doses of nasal decongestant medications may cause hypertension and a rapid heart rate because of their effect on arterioles throughout the body and stimulation of the heart, usually no significant rise in blood pressure occurs with their use. However, **when some cold medications are taken by mouth, they may significantly elevate blood pressure**, especially in hypertensives.

The NSAIDs are commonly used for arthritis and for relief of all sorts of pain. They include aspirin, Advil, Motrin, Nuprin, Indocin, Orudis, Naprosyn, Clinoril, Ansaid, Feldene, Voltaren, Celebrex, Aleve, and

Vioxx. **NSAIDs can interfere with antihypertensive treatment, and a significant increase in blood pressure may occur when these drugs are used chronically.** This hypertensive effect is reported to be less or insignificant with aspirin, Clinoril, Ansaid, Celebrex, and Vioxx. In contrast, blood pressure elevations are reported to be more pronounced with Indocin, Naprosyn, and ibuprofen-containing medications (such as Advil, Motrin, and Nuprin).

The elevation of blood pressure, which is only very rarely caused by NSAIDs, results when these substances inhibit the action of hormones (prostaglandins) that cause dilation of arterioles; this dilation is important for elimination of salt and water. The elderly, salt-sensitive patients, patients with impaired kidney function, and hypertensive patients all have a greater risk of developing severe hypertension or aggravating preexisting hypertension with the chronic use of NSAIDs because of excess retention of salt and water by the kidney. In addition, **NSAIDs can decrease the effectiveness of antihypertensive drugs and may occasionally cause ulcers in the stomach or intestine.** Although Tylenol does not affect blood pressure or cause ulcers, when it is taken in very large doses (for long periods) it may sometimes damage the kidneys and impair kidney function, thereby causing hypertension.

It is important to talk with your doctor about potential drug interactions and to learn which drugs to avoid if you have hypertension.

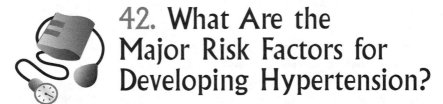

42. What Are the Major Risk Factors for Developing Hypertension?

Observations made at periodic intervals in a large number of people, including children, suggest that the major risk factors for developing hypertension are **a family history of hypertension in siblings or parents, excessive gain in weight, a rapid resting pulse rate, and a diet high in salt (sodium chloride) in those who are salt-sensitive.**

43. What Are the Major Risk Factors for Cardiovascular and Kidney Disease, and How Can I Reduce the Chances of These Complications?

Risk factors for heart disease (including heart attack and heart failure), stroke, transient ischemic attack (TIA), and kidney disease include the following:

- Hypertension
- Diabetes mellitus
- Cigarette smoking
- High LDL cholesterol ("bad" cholesterol)
- Low HDL cholesterol ("good" cholesterol)
- High triglycerides (blood fat)
- Family history of premature heart attack or stroke
- Sedentary lifestyle
- Obesity
- Older age
- For women, the postmenopausal state

For any level of blood pressure, the presence of one or more of these risk factors will increase the likelihood of a heart attack, heart failure, or stroke. Thus high blood pressure should be treated more aggressively in individuals who have additional risk factors than it is treated in those who do not have such risk factors. Treatment of high cholesterol levels with the goal of lowering LDL and raising HDL is equally important. Because age is also a risk factor (and one over which one has no control), elderly patients should receive aggressive treatment for high blood pressure and abnormal cholesterol levels, even if they do not have diabetes. Smoking cessation should be strongly urged, diabetes should be "tightly" controlled, and adequate exercise and a healthy diet should be included in your lifestyle (see Questions 44, 49, 51, 52, 62, 87, 89, 90, 95).

44. What Can I Do About Risk Factors If I Have Hypertension, and How Do They Affect Treatment?

Some risk factors for hypertension—age, gender, genetic, and racial background—obviously cannot be altered. In general, the risk of cardiovascular disease (heart attack, stroke, kidney and blood vessel damage) is greater in hypertensive men than in hypertensive women, and in African Americans than in white Americans, especially as people age. Until age 50, more men develop hypertension than women; however, after the menopause, women are more likely to develop hypertension than men of the same age. Hypertension occurs about twice as often in African Americans as in whites.

A history of premature cardiovascular disease in parents or siblings (that is, disease in men younger than 55 and women younger than 65 years old) confers an additional risk for cardiovascular complications. If one parent has essential hypertension, 25% of his or her children are predisposed to develop the condition; if both parents have hypertension, then roughly 75% of their offspring will become hypertensive (see Questions 11, 13, 26, 33).

The good news is that environmental risk factors for hypertension can be modified or eliminated:

- *Smoking cessation,* in addition to its many other benefits, will reduce the incidence of heart attacks and stroke and the damage to arteries caused by smoking (see Questions 51, 52).

- *Weight reduction* in individuals who are overweight will usually reduce hypertension and may help prevent development of hypertension (see Questions 47, 48, 49).

- *Curtailing excess salt consumption* can reduce and may help prevent hypertension in salt-sensitive individuals (see Question 34).

- *Reducing elevated LDL cholesterol* (low-density lipoprotein, the "bad" cholesterol) *and elevated triglyceride fats, and increasing HDL cholesterol* (high-density lipoprotein, the "good" cholesterol) can reduce damage to arteries and cardiovascular complications (see Questions 89, 90, 91).

- *Increasing exercise and avoiding a sedentary lifestyle* may lower elevated blood pressure, improve fitness of the heart, and aid in weight reduction (see Question 46).

- *Avoidance of excess alcohol consumption* may lower elevated blood pressure and does reduce the number of calories obtained from the alcohol, which may be very helpful in weight reduction (see Question 34).

- *Consumption of a diet low in saturated fat, high in fiber content, including liberal amounts of fruits and vegetables, and supplying lots of potassium* may not only lower blood pressure but also reduce the incidence of stroke (see Question 49).

Blood pressure control is of crucial importance in reducing the occurrence of cardiovascular complications. Consequently, all of the environmental factors mentioned above should be altered appropriately and medications utilized, if indicated. Finally, good control of diabetes is, of course, important in reducing some complications of diabetes.

Some risk factors for hypertension—age, gender, genetic, and racial background—obviously cannot be altered. The good news is that environmental risk factors can be modified or eliminated.

In 1997, the Sixth Joint National Committee Report (JNC VI) devised a strategy designed to improve the approach to treating hypertensive patients. The new approach considers not only the level of blood pressure elevation, but also any major risk factors and evidence of damage to various organs and arteries of the body (Table 5). Treatment is aimed at three risk groups and depends on the severity of the blood pressure elevation as well as the number of major risk factors and the amount of organ damage related to the hypertension.

- Risk Group A includes patients with high-normal blood pressure or stage 1, 2, or 3 hypertension (see Table 5) who do not have evidence of organ damage or other risk factors. Stage 1 patients may attempt to lower their blood pressure with lifestyle changes, plus close monitoring of their blood pressure. If blood pressure is not normalized in one year, then antihypertensive drug therapy should be added. For patients with stage 2 or 3 hypertension, drug and lifestyle changes are indicated.

- Risk Group B includes hypertensives who have no evidence of organ damage but one or more of the major risk factors (see Table 5) other than diabetes. This group accounts for the majority of hypertensive patients. If multiple risk factors are present, antihypertensive drugs and appropriate lifestyle modifications are indicated.

Table 5. *Strategy Recommended by the Sixth Joint National Committee Report (JNC VI) for Treating Hypertensive Patients*

Major risk factors	<ul><li>Cigarette smoking</li><li>Elevation of undesirable blood fats (LDL, triglycerides) and a decrease in desirable blood fats (HDL)</li><li>Diabetes</li><li>Age greater than 60 years</li><li>Being a man or a postmenopausal woman</li><li>Family history of premature cardiovascular disease (in women younger than 65 and men younger than 55 years old)</li></ul>
Evidence of organ damage	<ul><li>Heart disease — Enlargement of heart muscle of left ventricle (main pumping chamber) — Chest pain (angina) or previous heart attack — Prior angioplasty (balloon dilation) or coronary bypass surgery — Heart failure</li><li>Stroke or transient ischemic attack (TIA; ministroke)</li><li>Kidney damage</li><li>Damage to arteries (especially in the legs)</li><li>Damage to the retinal portion of the eye</li></ul>

Blood Pressure Classification	Systolic (mm Hg)		Diastolic (mm Hg)
Normal	Less than 130	and	Less than 85
High normal	Range 130–139	or	85–89
Stage 1	Range 140–159	or	90–99
Stage 2	Range 160–179	or	100–109
Stage 3	Greater than 179	or	Greater than 109

- Risk Group C consists of hypertensive patients who have diabetes or evidence of organ damage (see Table 5). These individuals (and some people with high-normal blood pressure as well as poor kidney function, heart failure, or diabetes) should be considered for prompt antihypertensive treatment plus appropriate lifestyle modifications.

Of paramount importance for the most successful management of patients with various degrees of hypertension is a careful assessment of the major risk factors and evidence of cardiovascular disease and organ damage. This information will help the physician in selecting the most appropriate treatment for each patient.

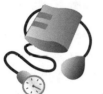

45. What Is Target Organ Disease, and How Does Its Presence Influence Treatment?

Target organ disease refers to disease in the organs that are most frequently damaged by high blood pressure—hence the term "target organs." The target organs of high blood pressure are the brain (strokes), the heart (heart attack and heart failure), the kidneys (kidney failure that may require dialysis), the eyes, and the arteries (arteriosclerosis or atherosclerosis). The presence of target organ damage is always a compelling reason to treat hypertension aggressively so as to protect these organs and prevent further damage (see Question 44).

46. What Are the Benefits of Exercise and Will It Lower My Blood Pressure?

Exercise is essential for your health and physical fitness (see Questions 40, 43, 60). Unfortunately, Americans have in recent years tended to be passive spectators rather than active participants in physical activities. For example, the advent of television has greatly eroded the time spent exercising. Sadly, our children are particularly obsessed with television and computers. One study of 10-year-old American girls revealed a direct correlation between excess body fat and hours spent watching TV. The increasing use of computers will merely compound the problem, further eroding participation in physical activity and reducing physical fitness. Only 22% of adults get at least 30 minutes of exercise during most days.

Sedentary persons are more likely to develop hypertension, heart attacks, and strokes than persons who are physically active. Regular, moderate aerobic exercise, on the other hand, can reduce both systolic and diastolic blood pressure in hypertensive subjects.

Sedentary persons ("couch potatoes") are more likely to develop hypertension, heart attacks, and strokes than persons who are physically active.

Furthermore, it has been demonstrated that regular, moderate aerobic exercise (that is, dynamic exercise that increases oxygen intake and increases activity of the heart, lungs, and muscles) can reduce systolic and diastolic blood pressure by about 10 and 8 mm Hg, respectively, in hypertensive subjects. It is noteworthy that moderate-intensity training appears to be just as effective as, if not better than, high-intensity exercise in providing many beneficial effects.

The benefits of regularly performing moderate aerobic exercise are many:

- Such exercise may prevent or minimize damage to the coronary arteries of the heart and improve heart function.

- Proper weight is more easily maintained.

- Muscle mass, strength, and agility are increased and preserved.

- Levels of the "good" blood cholesterol (HDL), which protects against hardening of the arteries, are increased, whereas levels of the "bad" cholesterol (LDL) and triglycerides (blood fats) are decreased.

- The risks of osteoporosis and diabetes are diminished.

- Emotional tension, anxiety, anger, and depression may be significantly alleviated.

Most recently, researchers have shown that exercise improves the ability of the heart arteries to dilate in response to a substance (nitric oxide) released from the lining of these arteries. This dilation occurs even in the presence of atherosclerosis (hardening of the arteries).

It is especially important to choose exercises that are enjoyable—if they are boring, it is almost certain that they will not be continued for very long. Exercise intensity and duration should be increased gradually and then performed for 30 or more minutes five or more times each week. Individuals older than 40 years, or anyone with any indication of heart or vascular disease, should consult a physician before embarking on an exercise program.

Walking and jogging are particularly popular types of exercise that can be performed alone, with a few friends, or in large groups. Bicycling, tennis, paddle tennis, squash, volleyball, cross-country skiing, skating, roller-blading, golf, swimming, aerobic group exercise, or dancing are all excellent ways of getting the exercise needed to improve cardiovascular fitness and muscle strength. Even regularly performed light-intensity exercise, such as Tai Chi, may reduce blood pressure modestly. Exercise machines (such as the treadmill, stationary bicycle, rowing machine, stair climber, and the vast array of dynamic muscle-building machines) are all excellent ways to work out and may be especially convenient; the opportunity to watch television, listen to music, or even read while using some of these machines can make the physical activity more enjoyable.* Most of these moderate-intensity exercises pose little chance of injury, especially if a few minutes of muscle stretching—a warm-up period—precedes the exercise.

Although exercise will transiently increase systolic pressure, systolic and diastolic pressures may be lower for as long as several hours after the activity ends. No evidence has been found to suggest that regular, moderate-intensity exercise increases the risk of stroke or heart attack in hypertensive individuals who have no heart disease or previous history of vascular disease of the brain. However, although lifting or "pressing" very heavy weights will build skeletal muscles, the straining required with isometrics (muscle contraction with little shortening but great increase in tone) should definitely be avoided. This type of activity can elevate both systolic and diastolic pressures, with systolic pressures sometimes reaching 300 mm Hg or higher! Repetitive, light weightlifting or exercises requiring intermittent contraction and relaxation of muscles, if not strenuous, are permissible. Severe elevations of blood pressure could be especially hazardous in persons using aspirin or anticoagulants.

Moderately intense exercise for 30 minutes will burn up approximately 150 calories. If it is more desirable to perform two 15-minute or three 10-minute periods of exercise, the benefits and total calories burned will be similar. Men burn up 10% to 20% more calories than women during exercise, probably due to men's greater muscle mass. One real benefit of physical activity is that, when combined with a reduced caloric intake, it can bring about significant weight loss and thereby further reduce blood pressure.

A good measure of fitness is your heart rate and length of time you can continue on a treadmill at different degrees of exercise. The maximum heart rate (pulse) you can achieve during exercise decreases with age. The pulse rate at your wrist or in your neck caused by exercising should be recorded (measure beats for 6 seconds immediately after exercise and multiply by 10 to calculate the beats per minute). With moderate exercise, this number should be roughly equivalent to 220 minus your age (the formula for maximum rate), multiplied by 70% (the recommended percentage of the maximum rate that should be attained during moderate exercise).

---

*One word of caution regarding the use of a Walkman if jogging or roller-blading on a road: The possibility of being hit by a car is increased if your hearing is impaired. Jogging or roller-blading is safer if done in the direction of oncoming cars, so that you can see and avoid them.

Most currently used antihypertensive medications do not interfere with the ability to exercise. Some drugs (beta blockers) that partially block the response of the heart to exercise, however, will limit the pumping action of the heart and slow the pulse. Consequently, these drugs may reduce a person's capacity for strenuous physical activity.

From the foregoing discussion, it should be obvious that the old adage "no pain, no gain" does not apply to exercise. Regularly performed, moderately intense exercise can be both very enjoyable and extremely beneficial to your health. So, if there are no medical contraindications, start exercising regularly and discover the many ways to enjoy it!

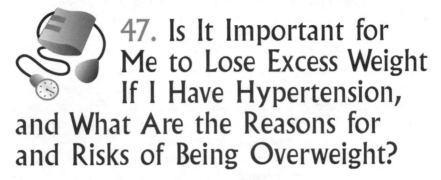

47. Is It Important for Me to Lose Excess Weight If I Have Hypertension, and What Are the Reasons for and Risks of Being Overweight?

If you are moderately overweight, your chance of having hypertension is three to six times greater than that of a healthy person with normal weight. If you are obese (that is, 20% or more above your ideal weight), your chance of developing hypertension may be as much as eight times greater than that of normal individuals; hypertension affects approximately 50% of obese individuals (see Questions 40, 42, 46).

If you are moderately overweight, your chance of having hypertension is three to six times greater than that of a healthy person with normal weight. If you are obese, your risk may be as much as eight times greater than that of normal individuals.

Obesity—defined as the excess accumulation of fat—is the most important environmental factor causing or aggravating hypertension. It may lead to retention of salt and water, constrict arterioles, and force the heart to pump harder. Loss of even 10 lb may significantly lower your elevated blood pressure. One study of obese hypertensive patients reported that the loss of 23 lb caused average systolic and diastolic pressures to decline by 11 and 8 mm Hg, respectively. If your blood pressure is borderline or minimally elevated, weight loss may return your pressure to normal and prevent the need for medication. In addition, weight loss may reduce the amount of antihypertensive medication that is required. Weight reduction can also lower your total cholesterol [particularly your low-density lipoprotein (LDL) cholesterol, which is the "bad" cholesterol] and decrease your risk of developing atherosclerosis (hardening of the arteries), heart attack, stroke, and diabetes.

Another reason for losing excess weight is that obesity predisposes a person to developing gallstones, degenerative arthritis, varicose veins and blood clots, toxemia of pregnancy, hernias, and (perhaps) breast, colon, uterus, gallbladder, and prostate cancer. Furthermore, in obese persons surgery is technically more difficult and complications of surgery are more frequent, wounds don't heal as fast, and infections are more common. These conditions usually account for the relatively high premature death rate associated with significant obesity. The more you weigh, the greater the risks.

Excess fat is a national health problem in the United States. Approximately 30% of all Americans are overweight, and another 25% are obese; that is, 55% of Americans are fat, more so than the percent of fat people in any other nation! Although the percentage of persons who are overweight has increased slightly in the last 40 years, the percentage who are obese has doubled! A simple way to determine ideal weight is the following:

- For men, use 106 lb for the first 5 feet, then add 6 lb for each additional inch of height.

- For women, use 100 lb for the first 5 feet, then add 5 lb for each additional inch of height.

A more accurate measure of ideal and excessive weight is body mass index (BMI), a weight-to-height index (Table 6). BMI can be determined by dividing your weight in kilograms by the square of your height in meters (kg/m^2). A BMI index of 19 to 24 is considered desirable, 25 to 29 indicates overweight, and over 30 indicates obesity. Table 7 conveniently presents height and weight standards for men and women of small, medium, and large frames (the weights of clothes and shoes were included).

Of particular interest is the fact that body shape of obese persons is a predictor of health risks. Fat that is confined mainly to the waist occurs more commonly in men and has been likened to an "apple shape"—a configuration that portends a higher risk for atherosclerosis, heart disease, hypertension, stroke, and diabetes. Fat in this area is metabolically very active; that is, it is released into the circulation and may accumulate in the arteries. A waist circumference of more than 40 inches in men, or 35 inches in women, is considered a health risk. If fat is mainly confined to the hips, buttocks, and thighs, imparting a "pear-shaped" body, then it appears to confer no greater health risks than in persons of normal weight. This configuration is seen more frequently in women. Fat in this location is metabolically inactive and does not cause arterial damage.

Table 6. What's Your Body Mass Index (BMI)?

Healthy		Overweight					Obesity				
BMI	19	24	25	26	27	28	29	30	35	40	45	50
Height					Weight in pounds							
4'10"	91	115	119	124	129	134	138	143	167	191	215	239
4'11"	94	119	124	128	133	138	143	148	173	198	222	247
5'0"	97	123	128	133	138	143	148	153	179	204	230	255
5'1"	100	127	132	137	143	148	153	158	185	211	238	264
5'2"	104	131	136	142	147	153	158	164	191	218	246	273
5'3"	107	135	141	146	152	158	163	169	197	225	254	282
5'4"	110	140	145	151	157	163	169	174	204	232	262	291
5'5"	114	144	150	156	162	168	174	180	210	240	270	300
5'6"	118	148	155	161	167	173	179	186	216	247	278	309
5'7"	121	153	159	166	172	178	185	191	223	255	287	319
5'8"	125	158	164	171	177	184	190	197	230	262	295	328
5'9"	128	162	169	176	182	189	196	203	236	270	304	338
5'10"	132	167	174	181	188	195	202	209	243	278	313	348
5'11"	136	172	179	186	193	200	208	215	250	286	322	358
6'0"	140	177	184	191	199	206	213	221	258	294	331	368
6'1"	144	182	189	197	204	212	219	227	265	302	340	378
6'2"	148	186	194	202	210	218	225	233	272	311	350	389
6'3"	152	192	200	208	216	224	232	240	279	319	359	399
6'4"	156	197	205	213	221	230	238	246	287	328	369	410

Source: Modified from National Institutes of Health. Clinical guidelines on the identification, evaluation and treatment of overweight and obesity in adults. Mayo Clinic on High Blood Pressure 1998.

In fewer than 5% of cases, obesity can be traced to hormonal disorders. Several factors are known to influence weight gain:

- *Genes* play a role in energy metabolism. With a family history of obesity, children have a 25% to 30% greater chance of being obese. Also, the weight of adopted children seems to correlate with the weight of their true parents rather than that of their foster parents.

- *Gender* also plays a role. For example, the greater muscle mass in men burns 10% to 20% more calories than in women at rest.

- *Aging* is accompanied by a decrease in muscle mass and a slowing of metabolism.

- *Overfeeding* in childhood may increase the number of fat cells and set the stage for lifelong obesity.

Table 7. Height and Weight Standards

Men				Women			
Height	*Small*	*Medium*	*Large*	*Height*	*Small*	*Medium*	*Large*
5'2"	128–134	131–141	138–150	4'10"	102–111	109–121	118–131
5'3"	130–136	133–143	140–153	4'11"	103–113	111–123	120–134
5'4"	132–138	135–145	142–156	5'0"	104–115	113–126	122–137
5'5"	134–140	137–148	144–160	5'1"	106–118	115–129	125–140
5'6"	136–142	139–151	146–164	5'2"	108–121	118–132	128–143
5'7"	138–145	142–154	149–168	5'3"	111–124	121–135	131–147
5'8"	140–148	145–157	152–172	5'4"	114–127	124–138	134–151
5'9"	142–151	148–160	155–176	5'5"	117–130	127–141	137–155
5'10"	144–154	151–163	158–180	5'6"	120–133	130–144	140–159
5'11"	146–157	154–166	161–184	5'7"	123–136	133–147	143–163
6'0"	149–160	157–170	164–188	5'8"	126–139	136–150	146–167
6'1"	152–164	160–174	168–192	5'9"	129–142	139–153	149–170
6'2"	155–168	164–178	172–197	5'10"	132–145	142–156	152–173
6'3"	158–172	167–182	176–202	5'11"	135–148	145–159	155–176
6'4"	162–176	171–187	181–207	6'0"	138–151	148–162	158–179

This table, which was developed by Metropolitan Life, shows desirable weight for size of frame for people 25 to 59 years old, in shoes with one-inch heels and wearing 5 lb of clothing for men and 3 lb of clothing for women.

- *Cessation of smoking* is accompanied by a reduced metabolic rate.
- *Physical inactivity* reduces energy expenditure, so that fewer calories are burned.
- *High-fat diets* increase weight by providing more calories than diets consisting mainly of protein and carbohydrate with limited fat. Even when calories are the same, however, more fat is stored in fat tissue when the diet is high in fat.

It is particularly noteworthy that some persons can significantly increase their consumption of calories without gaining weight, even though they do not increase their physical activity and energy expenditure. In these individuals, metabolism increases as their caloric intake increases.

Numerous endocrine and metabolic consequences of obesity have been identified. They account for the predisposition to diabetes and atherosclerosis. In particular, the four-element combination of obesity, diabetes, high levels of cholesterol and fat in the blood, and hypertension, has been dubbed "the deadly quartet" or "insulin resistance syndrome" (IRS). IRS appears to represent a syndrome (condition) of metabolic and endocrine disturbance marked by a decreased sensitivity to the metabolic action of insulin.

In 1994, Dr. J. M. Freedman and colleagues at Rockefeller University announced a most exciting discovery—a mutant or flawed gene linked to obesity in both rodents and humans. Strong experimental evidence suggests that a genetic mutation of the normally occurring obesity gene (the "Ob" gene) disrupts the body's energy metabolism and deranges the appetite control center in the brain. As a consequence, the signal for fullness or satiety is lost; overeating and weight gain then occur. This finding does not mean that obese persons cannot control their weight, if they desire to do so.

In the final analysis, obesity results from an excess consumption of calories and/or an insufficient expenditure of energy. Although the latter condition may result from lack of physical activity, energy expenditure also depends on body metabolism, which is genetically determined. You can't do anything about your genes, but you can control your weight by monitoring your eating habits and physical activity. It's up to you to take charge and protect your health by maintaining a normal weight!

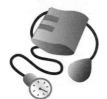

48. What Is the Best Way to Lose Excess Weight, and Are Diet Pills Indicated?

Persuading overweight and obese patients to reduce their weight is one of the most frustrating and difficult problems doctors face. Although doctors particularly recognize how important weight control is for the health of their patients (see Question 47), far too often patients seem unable to make a sustained commitment to reduce their weight, despite knowledge of health risks. **The single most important factor for a successful weight-loss program is the patient's motivation**. Effective treatment of excess weight or obesity is also fraught with frustration and emotional tension for patients. Americans spend more than $30 billion each year in trying to stay trim. Obviously, Americans find it very difficult to stay trim and thin, and to lose excess weight.

Altering lifestyle and eating patterns requires both mental and physical energy (see Questions 40, 46, 47). The combination of decreased caloric intake and increased caloric expenditure through increased physical activity with aerobic exercise (requiring active physical motion and increased oxygen consumption) is key to successful weight loss. Reducing the number of fatty meals and dairy products consumed is basic. Ideally, one should limit fat to no more than 30% of total calories in the diet.

The combination of decreased caloric intake and increased caloric expenditure through increased physical activity with aerobic exercise is key to successful weight loss.

Losing and regaining weight repeatedly ("yo-yo" dieting) may be hazardous—even resulting in higher death rates by increasing the risk of coronary artery disease. Severe dieting can lower the metabolic rate and cause the body to store fat faster and more effectively if one begins to eat more after the diet ends. As a consequence, such diets tend to cause people to regain even more weight.

Adequate exercise can prove very significant in preventing excess weight from recurring. Moderate or mild exercise—walking, golf, jogging, bicycling, tennis, swimming, cross-country skiing, calisthenics, dancing, exercise classes, or other activities—may be sufficient to keep the weight off, if the activity is performed several times weekly. Many individuals are most motivated to exercise when they take part in group activities. A brisk walk for 30 minutes four or five times each week should suffice. The type of exercise chosen should be enjoyable, because otherwise it may be discontinued.

Modest exercise can reduce weight and lower blood pressure just as effectively as strenuous exercise. Before embarking on any strenuous exercise program, the patient should consult a physician and obtain an electrocardiogram and stress test, if deemed necessary. To date, no evidence shows that vigorous exercise is more beneficial than regularly performed, moderate exercise. Aerobic exercise should be begun slowly, with the duration and intensity being gradually increased. There is no reason to perform strenuous isometric exercises such as heavy weightlifting, which is used to strengthen muscles and "body build," as this type of activity can raise blood pressure during exercise to dangerously high levels, especially in persons with hypertension.

It is noteworthy that men can eat more than women, because the greater muscle mass in men uses more energy. Under normal circumstances, men burn up 10% to 20% more calories than women. With aging and decrease in muscle mass, there is an accompanying decrease in metabolism, however.

Set a realistic goal for weight reduction, as an ideal weight can almost never be reached. A desirable goal is one that will reduce blood pressure, blood sugar, and cholesterol, if they are elevated. Gradual loss of weight (for example, 1 lb per week) is recommended, because this goal is attainable and such a pattern is most likely to succeed in permanent weight reduction. A simple way to determine how many calories you can eat daily and lose 1 lb each week is to multiply your weight in pounds by 10. For example, if you weigh 160 lb, 160 multiplied by 10 equals 1600 calories, which should be consumed daily to lose 1 lb per week.

To lose weight, it is very important to change your eating habits, to eat less, and to avoid excess calories and fat, which is so commonly consumed in the form of "fast foods." Consumption of lean meat, fish, chicken and turkey without the skin, and more grains, fruits and vegetables can offer an excellent balanced diet. Recently, the Dietary Approaches to Stop Hypertension (DASH) study demonstrated that a diet stressing fruits, vegetables, grains, and low-fat items (accounting for less than 30% of total calories) significantly reduced blood pressure in hypertensive patients and those with borderline elevations (see Question 49); it also promoted weight loss. This diet was rich in potassium, calcium, and magnesium, and potassium probably played a role in lowering blood pressure. The evidence showing the ability of dietary calcium and magnesium to lower elevated blood pressure was not as convincing, however.

Consumption of lean meat, fish, chicken and turkey without the skin, and more grains, fruits and vegetables can offer an excellent balanced diet.

Increased consumption of water, nonfattening beverages, and high-fiber foods may help curb the appetite. "Snacking" between meals must be avoided; it may help to eat carrot and celery sticks if the urge to snack arises. Alcohol consumption in men should be limited to no more than 2 oz of whiskey, 10 oz (2 wine glasses) of wine, or 24 oz (2 cans) of beer daily; women and thin persons should consume even less alcohol. Alcohol is a source of non-nutritional calories, which can add to weight problems; furthermore, exceeding the recommended limits can increase blood pressure. It has been reported that excessive alcohol consumption may account for the elevated blood pressure in 7% to 10% of the hypertensive population.

"Crash diets" involving special food combinations, liquid drinks, and packaged foods, as well as very-low-calorie diets, are not recommended, because they may prove hazardous and are usually ineffective for long-term weight loss. A healthy diet consists of 30% or less fat, about 60% carbohydrate with very little refined sugar, and about 10% protein.

Dr. Robert Atkins advocates the use of diets high in protein and fat and low in carbohydrates (that is, no more than 20% of total calories) for weight reduction. Although this diet can curb the appetite, reduce caloric intake, cause weight loss, and even lower blood cholesterol in some people, many find it very difficult to adhere to a low-carbohydrate diet. Such a diet bans fruit and fruit juice, bread, grains, potato, rice, corn, dairy products (other than cheese, cream, or butter) and sugar in any form. Weight loss may fail to occur, and cholesterol levels may increase significantly, if carbohydrates are not strictly limited. It is noteworthy that most Asians are not obese, yet consume diets high in carbohydrates.

Dr. Dean Ornish advocates an almost fat-free diet—similar to a strict vegetarian diet—for weight loss. Many individuals cannot adhere to this diet, however, and vitamin and iron deficiency may occur without proper supplementation of these substances.

Over-the-counter appetite suppressants should be used with caution. They can stimulate the nervous system and may increase blood pressure; in addition, they do not suppress appetites for long periods of time. One setback in the search for an effective appetite suppressant occurred in 1997. At that time, it was reported that the appetite suppressant "fen-phen"—the combination of fenfluramine (Pondimin) or dexfenfluramine (Redux) with phentermine—caused thickening and sometimes malfunctioning of heart valves on the left side of the heart in an alarming number of patients consuming this drug for weight reduction (6 million Americans had used fen-phen). Some patients also developed increased blood pressure in the lung, which sometimes proved fatal. As a consequence of these side effects, use of these drugs was discontinued.

Recently, orlistat (Xenical), which prevents absorption of 30% of dietary fat, has been approved by the U.S. Food and Drug Administration for long-term treatment of obesity. This drug should be considered as an aid for some obese patients who are resistant to weight-loss programs, especially those individuals with hypertension, diabetes, and/or elevated fats in their blood. It is recommended that orlistat be taken three times daily with each meal containing fat; it can be omitted if the meal does not include fat. **Orlistat appears modestly effective in promoting weight loss and should be considered in some very obese patients; however, it frequently causes bloating, flatulence, oily stools, diarrhea and fecal urgency, and incontinence.** Furthermore, it interferes with the absorption of the fat-soluble vitamins A, D, E, and K and beta-carotene; replacement of fat-soluble vitamins, with the supplements being consumed two hours before or after orlistat, is indicated in patients taking orlistat. The side effects associated with this drug may be minimized by reducing fat in the diet. Orlistat should not be taken by patients who have any type of intestinal disease that prevents food/nutrition absorption, and it should not be used during pregnancy or by nursing mothers.

As a last resort, in some very obese individuals who are unable to lose weight, surgical procedures to reduce the amount of food absorbed from the intestine have been performed; however, this procedure is rarely recommended.

Weight reduction can do wonders for your physical and mental health, and it may also improve your energy level. Motivation and commitment to a weight-loss program, of course, are essential ingredients for success. It's up to you!

49. What Is the Best Diet to Treat Hypertension and Its Complications? What Are the "Mediterranean" and "DASH" Diets?

The best diet for a person with hypertension satisfies the following criteria:

- It allows the person to avoid becoming overweight or obese, and it maintains weight near the normal acceptable standard range.
- It limits total salt (sodium chloride) intake to no more than 6 grams (g) (about one teaspoonful) daily (equivalent to 2400 milligrams of sodium).
- It limits alcohol consumption to no more than two drinks of wine, beer, or spirits per day.
- It helps lower "bad" cholesterol (LDL—low-density lipoprotein) and fat (triglyceride) levels, if they are elevated.
- It includes food with minerals (potassium) that tend to lower blood pressure.

The importance of losing excess body weight for hypertensive patients and the best means of losing weight are discussed in detail elsewhere in this book (see Questions 47, 48). Here, we emphasize once again that weight loss is best achieved by reducing caloric consumption (with less than 30% fat in the diet) and by increasing caloric expenditure through regular, moderate exercise performed for 30 minutes four or five times per week. Reducing the total number of calories in the diet is essential and can be achieved by reducing fat consumption: 1 g of fat is equivalent to 9 calories, whereas 1 g of protein or carbohydrate is equivalent to only 4 calories. Weight loss of even a few pounds may reduce blood pressure. Indeed, weight loss is certainly one of the most effective ways of reducing blood pressure without drugs.

Restricting total salt (sodium chloride) consumption to no more than 6g (one teaspoonful) per day can also reduce blood pressure in hypertensive individuals who are salt-sensitive—that is, those who develop hypertension when they consume excess amounts of salt (see Question 34). This group may account for 50% to 60% of the hypertensive population. Most African Americans are especially sensitive to salt. Approximately 75% of salt consumed comes from processed food (that is, food prepared by a food company for public consumption). Only a relatively small percentage is found in unprocessed food (that is, naturally occurring food to which nothing has been added), and only 15% is usually added to the cooking or at the table. It is especially important to read food labels and become aware of foods that have a high concentration of sodium so that you can avoid them. Even some local water supplies may have a high content of sodium.

Cardia is an acceptable salt substitute, as it contains much less sodium than normal salt. It also contains potassium and magnesium, which may even aid in lowering blood pressure. Nevertheless, any salt substitute containing potassium should be used with caution in individuals with impaired kidney function, as retention of excessive amounts of potassium can damage the electrical impulses and function of the heart. Potassium-containing salt substitutes should not be used in individuals receiving a potassium-sparing diuretic, as their consumption could elevate potassium in the blood to harmful levels. Fruits and vegetables are an excellent source of potassium.

Potassium-containing salt substitutes should be used with caution in individuals with impaired kidney function and should not be used at all in individuals receiving a potassium-sparing diuretic.

Excessive alcohol consumption is responsible for hypertension in 7% to 10% of all cases (see Question 24). This hypertension appears to result from stimulation of the brain and nervous system, which in turn causes constriction of the arterioles. Women with hypertension should consume less alcohol than hypertensive men, because women are usually smaller and metabolize alcohol less efficiently than men do. It should be appreciated that alcohol adds calories to the diet, which is undesirable for a person who is trying to lose weight. Some evidence, however, suggests that limited alcohol consumption actually protects individuals from heart attacks and damage to arteries of the heart when compared to those who do not drink alcohol. The beneficial effect conferred by consumption of modest amounts of alcohol seems to result from improvements in cholesterol concentrations; alcohol may slightly increase good cholesterol (HDL—high-density lipoprotein) levels.

Elevation of "bad" cholesterol (LDL) levels and probably elevation of triglyceride (another lipid) levels in the blood increase the risk of heart attacks, strokes, and hardening of the arteries. In the presence of hypertension, the risk of these complications is significantly increased, which makes it even more important to reduce the level of these fats in addition to normalizing blood pressure.

Reduction of "bad" cholesterol and triglycerides may be accomplished in several ways:

- Reduced consumption of dietary cholesterol and fats (by limiting consumption of fat to no more than 30% of caloric intake)

- Weight reduction, if overweight

- Taking cholesterol- and fat-lowering drugs, if indicated

One should be aware of foods containing cholesterol and harmful fats, especially saturated fats (animal fats, lard, dairy products, chocolate, coconut and palm oil, and some vegetable shortening), and trans-fatty acids (present in margarine and in crackers, cookies, and cakes). These fats should be avoided but can be replaced when necessary with monounsaturated fats, particularly olive oil. It is noteworthy that people in Spain, France, Italy, and Greece, who tend to consume lots of olive oil, vegetables, fruits, and grains but little saturated fat and processed foods (known as the "Mediterranean diet"), have relatively little heart disease. Polyunsaturated fats, such as corn, sunflower, safflower, and soybean oils, are also far healthier than saturated fats. Nevertheless, all oils are fats and can add a significant amount of calories if used too much. If weight loss and diet are unable to sufficiently lower LDL cholesterol and triglycerides, then drug treatment may be indicated.

Recently, the Dietary Approaches to Stop Hypertension (DASH) diet has been found to be effective in lowering blood pressure in hypertensive individuals (see Questions 48, 97). This diet has also been recommended as a very healthy diet for all Americans. The DASH diet consists of 27% calories from fat, lots of fruits and vegetables (8 to 10 servings daily), low-fat or nonfat dairy products, nuts, grains, fiber, and small amounts of

The DASH diet has been found to be effective in lowering blood pressure in hypertensive individuals and has been recommended as a very healthy diet for all Americans.

meat, fish, and poultry. After eight weeks on the DASH diet, the systolic and diastolic pressures in hypertensive individuals participating in the study decreased by 11.4 and 5.5 mm Hg, respectively. Even persons with high-normal blood pressures experienced a decrease of about 3.5 mm Hg in their systolic pressure and 2 mm Hg in their diastolic pressure. Diets rich in fruits and vegetables but higher in fat also decreased blood pressure, albeit less dramatically than the DASH diet did. On the other hand, researchers did not observe any change in blood pressure of individuals on the typical American diet, which contains approximately 37% of calories in the form of fat and is low in fruits and vegetables. In the study, the salt content remained the same in all diets (about 7.5 g of salt) and all diets contained the same number of calories (about 2000). The significant decrease in blood pressure found with the DASH diet occurred without any other lifestyle changes, which indicates the value of decreasing fat and increasing consumption of minerals, which are abundant in fruits and vegetables.

Experimental and clinical studies suggest that increased consumption of potassium is valuable in gradually reducing blood pressure and preventing stroke. The potassium content of the DASH diet is roughly 2½ times that consumed in an ordinary diet in the United States.

The roles played by other minerals in fruits and vegetables (such as calcium and magnesium) and by fat reduction in decreasing blood pressure are less clear. It appears that some salt-sensitive hypertensives who are calcium-deficient may lower their blood pressure by consuming additional calcium, which may increase salt and water excretion. Potentially, the DASH diet could actually prevent hypertension in some individuals. At any rate, the DASH diet is an extremely healthy diet, which should be recommended to all Americans. For individuals with high blood pressure, however, we recommend that salt be limited to 6 g daily instead of the 7.5 g in the DASH diet.

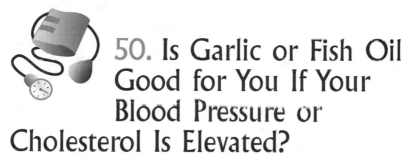

50. Is Garlic or Fish Oil Good for You If Your Blood Pressure or Cholesterol Is Elevated?

Any food purported to benefit persons with hypertension or high levels of blood cholesterol should have its claims validated by scientific evaluation before the medical profession advises its use or the public accepts it. The claims of the beneficial effects from many "health foods" are unsubstantiated and fraudulent, and their consumption may result in an enormous financial investment without any reward.

Although the beneficial effects of garlic on blood pressure and cholesterol were controversial and inconclusive for many years, more recently several studies involving about 1000 persons reported that taking 600 to 1000 milligrams (mg) daily of garlic supplements lowered total cholesterol by 9% to 12%. Consumption of garlic also caused levels of triglycerides (another fat in the blood, which may be harmful) to decrease, but "good" cholesterol (HDL—high-density lipoprotein) remained unchanged. Furthermore, it has been reported that even 500 mg of garlic supplements taken daily for seven years protected arteries from becoming stiff and hardened by deposits of cholesterol when compared to the arteries of those not taking the garlic. Some believe that raw garlic cloves are more effective than the supplements. Allicin, an oil in garlic, appears to be responsible for lowering cholesterol in the blood.

Garlic supplements appear to lower total cholesterol and triglycerides, but do not affect "good" (HDL) cholesterol levels.

In the past few years, several studies have reported that garlic—usually in the form of deodorized powder—lowers blood pressure. In one study, systolic blood pressure decreased by 11 mm Hg when subjects took such supplements. Unfortunately, a considerable amount of raw or deodorized powdered garlic (available in capsules dispensed as Kwai) must be consumed daily to lower blood pressure. Furthermore, a recent extensive review of studies on the therapeutic values of garlic indicates that **garlic does not have any antihypertensive action**. Other ways of lowering cholesterol and blood pressure are much more effective, reliable, and practical. Consequently, garlic is not prescribed by physicians to treat hypertension or elevated cholesterol. Garlic can inhibit blood clotting and may augment the effect of anticoagulants.

Onions come from the same vegetable family as garlic and have been reported to have similar therapeutic benefits. Nevertheless, the amounts ordinarily consumed do not provide any significant beneficial effects on blood pressure or cholesterol.

A few years ago, considerable excitement was generated by reports that fish oil was good for lowering cholesterol and blood pressure and would protect against heart attack. Eskimos, who eat large amounts of fish, whale, and seal meat (all of which contain lots of fish oil), have relatively low total cholesterol and triglycerides in their blood and a decreased tendency for their blood to clot. In addition, Eskimos have significantly fewer heart attacks than non-Eskimos who do not consume a diet high in fish oil. As a result of the enthusiastic reports regarding the beneficial effects of fish oil, the sale of fish oil capsules soared to $45 million in one year.

Fish oil contains omega-3 polyunsaturated fatty acids, which occur naturally in fish and are especially abundant in tuna, mackerel, trout, and salmon. Such fatty acids are important in forming chemicals in humans that can lower cholesterol and triglycerides and can increase "good" cholesterol (HDL). They also exert a mild effect in preventing blood from clotting, and they form substances that can lower blood pressure by dilating arteries. All of these effects of omega-3 fatty acids would tend to prevent damage to arteries and would reduce the likelihood of heart attacks and strokes.

Fish oil capsules are available in several commercial preparations. Large doses, however, are required to produce a beneficial effect on blood pressure and blood triglycerides; little or no change occurs in the "bad" cholesterol (LDL). Unfortunately, very large doses have been linked to a greater risk of bleeding, and the high concentrations of vitamin A and D contained in fish oil can be toxic. Capsules of fish oil are, of course, high in fat and calories—characteristics that are undesirable if you are trying to lose weight—and they may cause intestinal upset and have an unpleasant, fishy after-taste. In fact, it appears that eating fish several times per week may be just as effective in lowering blood pressure and reducing levels of cholesterol and fats in the blood as consuming capsules of fish oil. In one study, eating two cans of mackerel daily for two weeks decreased systolic and diastolic blood pressure by 15 and 7 mm Hg, respectively, decreased total cholesterol by 7% and triglycerides by 50%, and increased "good" cholesterol (HDL).

The American Heart Association and experts managing hypertension and cholesterol and fat abnormalities in the blood have concluded that eating fish several times each week may reduce the risk of vascular disease and possibly protect against heart attack and stroke. **Because large doses of omega-3 fatty acids are required for any beneficial therapeutic effect, and because toxic side effects are possible, prolonged use of supplements is not recommended**. Frequent consumption of fish, however, is highly desirable.

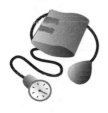

51. Must I Give Up Smoking Because of My Hypertension?

The answer to this question is an emphatic "yes"! There is no more treacherous contributor to health problems than cigarette smoking. Even smoke from cigars or pipes is hazardous to your health. The havoc caused by smoking is monumental, and it is the most preventable cause of premature death in the United States. It causes more than 1100 deaths per day and 20% of all deaths, and smoking-related medical care costs approximately $50 billion annually. In addition, 15% of persons who smoke cigarettes develop lung cancer.

Smoking accounts for several alarming statistics:

- 30% of cardiovascular deaths (including heart attack, heart failure, stroke, and blood vessel damage)
- 30% of all cancer deaths (including 87% of lung cancer deaths)
- 80% of deaths from chronic obstructive lung disease (primarily emphysema)

Consider this sobering fact: Smoking cigarettes causes lung and laryngeal cancer, chronic bronchitis, coronary heart disease, hardening of the arteries (atherosclerosis), cancer of the mouth and esophagus, chronic obstructive lung disease, low-birth-weight babies, unsuccessful pregnancies, increased infant mortality, and peptic ulcer. It may be a contributing factor for development of cancer of the urinary bladder, pancreas, kidneys, and stomach. In addition, smoking appears to be associated with stroke and possibly cataracts, bowel disease, macular degeneration, and breast cancer. It can decrease the "good" cholesterol (HDL) and increase the "bad" cholesterol (LDL) in your blood. It may also cause platelets (small blood cells) to aggregate and form clots that could block the circulation and cause a heart attack or stroke.

Smoking a pipe or cigars may be less injurious to a person's health than inhaling cigarette smoke. Nevertheless, these forms of smoking still pose a significant risk not only to the smoker, but also to all those who inhale the smoke passively.

The nicotine in cigarettes increases your heart rate and constricts your blood vessels, which may raise your blood pressure for 30 to 60 minutes. Roughly one-third of all hypertensives smoke. Nicotine is believed to lessen the effectiveness of some antihypertensive drugs, particularly the beta blockers. Although smoking does not cause permanent hypertension, the repeated transient elevations of blood pressure associated with it may prove harmful.

Dr. Tom Pickering, using ambulatory blood pressure monitoring for 24 hours, demonstrated that, during the day, systolic pressures were 5 to 10 mm Hg higher in one-pack-a-day smokers than in nonsmokers; at night, no such difference in pressures was noted between smokers and nonsmokers. Based on his findings, smoking even one pack per day appears to be responsible for a mildly elevated blood pressure in normal healthy subjects—clearly demonstrating the effect of nicotine. It seems reasonable to suggest that this daytime, smoking-related increase would augment the blood pressure of hypertensive individuals and possibly increase their risk of complications.

Nicotine activates the sympathetic nervous system and releases hormones (adrenaline and noradrenaline) into the circulation that not only increase your heart rate and blood pressure, but may also cause irregular heart beats. In addition, smoking decreases the supply of oxygen to tissues and vital organs. It adds carbon monoxide to the blood, which may damage blood vessels, permit cholesterol accumulation in the arteries, and accelerate atherosclerosis. Indeed, the arteries of the heart (coronary arteries) are more frequently and more severely damaged in smokers than they are in nonsmokers.

Although heavy or chain smokers are at greater risk than light smokers for developing the diseases mentioned above, nonsmokers who are exposed to cigarette smoke from others (from "passive smoking") are also at increased risk for heart and lung disease. It has been reported that persons living with a smoker have a 30% greater chance of developing heart disease than if they were not exposed to smoke. Such passive smoking is estimated to cause 37,000 deaths yearly. Children of parents who smoke are also more likely to suffer from lung infections and asthma than children who are not exposed to smoke.

Cigarette smokers without any health problems are two to three times more likely to have a heart attack than nonsmokers, and the odds of surviving a heart attack are usually worse in those who smoke. The presence of high blood pressure, elevated blood cholesterol, diabetes, or obesity all further increase the risk of heart attack, stroke, and blood vessel damage (hardening of the arteries with a blockage and/or rupture of these vessels). Smokers with hypertension are three to five times more likely to die from a heart attack or heart failure than nonsmokers and twice as likely to die of a stroke. As the number of risk factors increases, so too does the risk of premature death; with each additional risk factor, the chance of death may double. If all risk factors are present, the chance of premature death is enormous.

The good news is that 40 million Americans have given up smoking, and it is extremely rare to see a physician who smokes. Unfortunately, 50 million Americans continue to smoke. Sadly, the number of teenagers who smoke is increasing—especially young women. Psychosocial (that is, emotional and social experiences) and peer pressures play a central role in influencing the attitudes of many teenagers. Some young women apparently use cigarettes to stay slim, as smoking increases body metabolism and can curb the appetite (see Question 52).

Additional good news is that one year after cessation of smoking, the risk of cardiovascular disease diminishes markedly; the risk of heart disease decreases by approximately 50%, and five years after smoking cessation it is almost the same as in nonsmokers. The risk of lung and other cancers, strokes, and chronic lung disease decrease as well. After 10 to 15 years of abstinence, it has been reported that the risk of death from a smoking-related disease is nearly as low as that of persons who never smoked.

Cessation of cigarette smoking is the most effective and important life insurance policy available. For your sake and for the health of your family and all those with whom you come in contact, give it up!

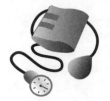

52. What Is the Best Way to Quit Smoking?

With any form of addiction, whether it be addiction to alcohol, drugs, or cigarette smoking, *motivation* is absolutely essential in quitting. Without

> **With any form of addiction, whether it be addiction to alcohol, drugs, or cigarette smoking, motivation *is* absolutely essential in quitting.**

sufficient commitment to abstain, the smoking cessation plan has little, if any, chance of success. To underscore the importance of motivation, note that 95% of the 40 million persons who have quit smoking have done it on their own. The poor success rates of many formal smoking cessation programs are most likely related to insufficient motivation (see Question 51).

It is usually not easy to quit smoking, especially for the heavy smoker, because most smokers are physically and psychologically addicted. However, the fear of disease caused by cigarette smoking has very significantly affected Americans, and tobacco consumption has decreased by 25% during the past 20 years. Today, it is extremely rare for U.S. physicians to smoke, because they are acutely aware of the habit's enormous and serious health risks. Many people in this country are aware that even the male model used in one of the Marlboro cigarette ads died of lung cancer. Unfortunately, the seriousness of the health hazards of smoking has not been sufficiently transmitted to populations outside of the United States, where smoking remains prevalent at all levels of society and in all professions.

Millions of Americans try to give up smoking each year, but only 10% are successful on the first attempt. Persistence plus firm motivation are the keys to success. Nearly two-thirds of all people who repeatedly try to quit eventually succeed. Also, it is never too late to quit, given that health benefits may be gained by abstaining from this habit, no matter what the age of the individual and how long the duration of cigarette smoking.

There is no magic formula for smoking cessation. Some smokers will respond to one approach better than another. Although smoking is physically addictive due to the activity of nicotine, it also results in strong psychological and social dependence because it becomes associated with a large variety of situations and emotional states. Stressful situations may be lessened and concentration improved by smoking, which makes it especially desirable under some circumstances. Repeatedly smoking at a particular time of the day, under a large variety of emotionally stressful circumstances, and during special social events and periods of entertainment can cause the habit to become ingrained and trigger the desire to automatically smoke at these times.

For smoking cessation to be most successful, certain steps should be followed. Deviation from these guidelines may be desired by some smokers, however, and may not doom the effort to quit.

First and foremost, an earnest desire to quit smoking is essential. One should be prepared to experience short-term discomfort (irritability, anxiety, and loss of concentration), which becomes most noticeable 2 to 4 days after cessation but usually disappears within 10 to 14 days. Thereafter, the desire to smoke may periodically occur months or years later, but this urge to smoke usually lasts only a few seconds. It is extremely important to appreciate that anyone who has been a heavy smoker cannot become a "social smoker." Any "slip"—even smoking one cigarette—is very likely to cause full resumption of smoking (much like the case with former chronic alcoholics or former cocaine or heroine addicts). Relapses are most apt to occur during negative emotional states within the first few months after quitting.

In general, the following suggestions and approach to smoking cessation have proved helpful:

1. **Consider the importance of quitting and list the health hazards of smoking and the important reasons you wish to quit.** Enlist the help of others—especially your family and friends—to give moral support and ask them to avoid smoking in your presence. Make a list of locations and situations when you are most apt to smoke, and be prepared to either avoid these circumstances or cope with them. Each day check the reasons you want to quit. Then designate a date on which to quit, preferably a day when your stress level is low and you face few problems and pressures.

2. **Stopping abruptly seems to be more effective than trying to cut down gradually.** Throw away all cigarettes and matches. The use of Zyban (bupropion, Wellbutrin), an antidepressant, has proved especially valuable in some smokers because this drug reduces the desire to smoke, even in persons who are not depressed. Zyban may be effective alone, but is more commonly used in conjunction with nicotine replacement. It requires a prescription and the dosage and schedule for use should be left to your physician.

Nicotine replacement may be especially helpful in heavy smokers who are addicted. Nicotine transdermal patches (such as Habitrol, Nicoderm, and Prostep) offer significant advantages over nicotine chewing gum (Nicorette): the former products are easier to use, cause fewer side effects, and deliver a more constant and adequate dose of nicotine. Although nicotine patches can be purchased without a prescription, you should consult with your physician regarding dosage schedules, especially when the patches are used in combination with Zyban. Other forms of nicotine delivery—by means of a nasal spray or inhaler, for example—appear to be much less effective than patches and chewing gums containing nicotine.

You must not smoke if you are using nicotine replacement, because smoking might significantly elevate the nicotine concentration in the blood and cause problems, especially in individuals with heart disease. Anecdotal reports suggesting that nicotine patches may cause heart irregularities and even heart attacks or strokes have raised concern; a study of male volunteers, however, revealed no differences in side effects between subjects using nicotine patches and those using patches without nicotine.

The value of hypnosis and acupuncture is poorly substantiated as a means of smoking cessation, although some have benefited from these treatments.

3. **Be prepared to cope with the urge to smoke, which is especially strong initially during withdrawal symptoms.** Changing routine activities may be very helpful. Avoid locations and situations where you routinely smoke. Perform activities to divert your attention such as exercising, taking a walk immediately after meals, going to a movie, joining friends who are strongly opposed to smoking, chewing ordinary gum, eating celery, carrot sticks, or unsalted pretzels, and sucking on Tic-Tacs. You should avoid substituting high-calorie foods for cigarettes, because smoking cessation decreases the body's metabolism and leads to a tendency to gain weight. Continually recall the health hazards of smoking, including death from heart and lung disease, stroke, a variety of cancers, and risks to the fetus during pregnancy.

Some smokers may be helped by formal cessation programs with group interaction and mutual support. You must always remember that the key to quitting depends almost entirely on the strength of your desire to quit! **If you fail to quit on the first attempt, always try again.** You may learn from failure how to be successful. It is worth repeating that two-thirds of those who repeatedly try to quit eventually succeed.

53. Are Atherosclerosis and Arteriosclerosis the Same? What Are Their Complications and Can They Cause Hypertension?

Although technical differences exist between atherosclerosis and arteriosclerosis (commonly called hardening of the arteries), for practical purposes they are the same—and both are treacherous. These conditions can lead to blockage of the arteries (heart attacks and strokes), kidney disease, amputations (especially of the lower extremities), and aneurysms (weakened areas in the arterial wall that expand like a balloon and sometimes rupture). Both atherosclerosis and arteriosclerosis are aggravated by high blood pressure, high blood cholesterol, and cigarette smoking. They are particularly common in countries where consumption of dairy and animal products is high and where hypertension is common.

For practical purposes, atherosclerosis and arteriosclerosis are the same—and both are treacherous. These conditions can lead to blockage of the arteries, kidney disease, amputations, and aneurysms.

Reducing blood pressure, lowering cholesterol, and stopping smoking will slow down the sclerotic process. People who do not have diabetes, high blood pressure, or high cholesterol, and who do not smoke cigarettes, rarely have atherosclerosis or arteriosclerosis in any form.

With the modern diets typical of industrialized societies, hardening of the arteries occurs with aging and results in increased systolic pressure (see Questions 22 and 37). Over time, the large arteries become hardened and lose much of their elasticity, causing increased resistance to the blood expelled by the heart during contraction (systole). Hardening of the arteries supplying the kidneys can sometimes significantly impair blood flow to the kidneys, which may then release renin. The renin is converted to angiotensin, a hormone that causes constriction of arterioles and thereby leads to hypertension (see Question 38).

54. Should High Blood Pressure Be Treated Differently in Men and Women, and in African Americans and White Individuals?

Prior to beginning menopause, women are less likely than men of comparable age to be hypertensive, and their risk of heart attack and stroke

None of the drugs that lower blood pressure appears to be more effective in one gender than in the other.

is less than that in men of comparable age. After menopause, however, the protective effect of estrogen is lost. Consequently, the frequency of high blood pressure is as great, if not greater, in postmenopausal women than in men of comparable age. Furthermore, elderly women have as many heart attacks and strokes as do elderly men. For these reasons, **it is important to treat high blood pressure in men and women of any age,** and to seek out and treat other risk factors for cardiovascular disease such as cigarette smoking, diabetes mellitus, and high cholesterol. No convincing evidence exists to suggest that any of the drugs that lower blood pressure are more effective in one gender than in the other.

It is well established that African Americans—both men and women—are more likely to have hypertension than white individuals. Hypertension is also more likely to be severe in African Americans than it is in whites, leading to complications at an earlier age in African Americans (see Question 26). Consequently, this condition should be treated equally as aggressively in both African Americans and whites. Young African American men are particularly vulnerable to developing the devastating consequences of high blood pressure. Because they do not consult a physician as frequently as whites of the same age, their hypertension may go undiscovered and untreated.

For both men and women, diuretics and calcium-blocking drugs seem to be more effective in African Americans and older subjects than are other drugs, although some African Americans respond well to ACE inhibitors, angiotensin II receptor blockers, and beta blockers. For some patients of either gender or race, multiple drugs may be necessary to control hypertension, especially when it is severe.

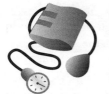

55. Once I Start Taking Medicine for High Blood Pressure, Do I Have to Take It Forever?

Usually you have to take antihypertensive drugs on a continuing basis, if you want your blood pressure to remain normal. Medication to lower blood pressure controls but does not cure hypertension. In this sense, hypertension is analogous to diabetes. Patients with diabetes must take pills or insulin to maintain their blood sugar in a normal range, but the therapy does not cure the diabetes. Similarly, medication controls hypertension only so long as you take the drugs.

Occasionally, patients who keep their blood pressures well controlled with medication for more than two years will be able to gradually reduce the dose taken without any rise in blood pressure. This is particularly true for patients who modify their lifestyle so as to lose excess weight and then remain lean, exercise regularly, and consume very little salt. Most of the time, however, when patients stop taking their antihypertensive medications, their blood pressure returns to the original, higher level. It may take days, weeks, or months for this increase to occur, depending upon how long blood pressure has been adequately controlled. With prolonged use of a drug to control blood pressure, the return of pressure to the formerly elevated level may take longer than if the medication was used for only a short period and then discontinued. If side effects are a reason for discontinuing the medication, you should consult with your doctor—a different medication may be just as effective and offer few adverse effects.

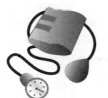

56. Can Caffeine Be Harmful and Should I Give It Up If I Have Hypertension?

Consumption of coffee and tea is almost a ritual in practically all cultures and countries throughout the world. This ingrained behavior often adds to the zest of life, offering an opportunity for repeated social communication among friends and fellow workers. Many find it difficult and unpleasant to start the morning without coffee. Although the exhilaration of caffeine can account for some of this physical caffeine dependence, coffee drinking also provides psychological support to many. Children do not, of course, share this need for morning coffee, but they may consume excess amounts of caffeine in soft drinks and chocolate to the point of causing nervousness, irritability, and difficulty in relaxing. Coffee is a very important part of most adult lives, and it has been estimated that one-half of the U.S. population drinks three or more cups of coffee each day!

Table 8 lists the concentration of caffeine in coffee, tea, soft drinks, chocolate, and "decaffeinated" drinks. In most people, caffeine increases alertness, concentration, and job performance, and it can lift one's mood. This effect may be accompanied by a *temporary* increase in heart rate and blood pressure in both hypertensive and normotensive persons. One cup of strong coffee may increase diastolic blood pressure by 8 mm Hg in men with mild hypertension, whereas an increase of 3 mm Hg may occur in individuals with normal blood pressure. Furthermore, excess caffeine consumption can cause nervousness, irritability, anxiety, shakiness, panic attacks, insomnia, and inability to relax and concentrate. If you want to decrease excessive caffeine consumption, proceed gradually so as to prevent headaches and other side effects that may result from reducing caffeine intake suddenly.

> *Excess caffeine consumption can cause nervousness, irritability, anxiety, shakiness, panic attacks, insomnia, and inability to relax and concentrate. It may also produce a temporary increase in heart rate and blood pressure in both hypertensive and normotensive persons.*

To date, little evidence has been found to suggest that the constriction of blood vessels due to caffeine consumption damages arteries or leads to heart attacks or strokes. Because caffeine stimulates the heart muscle and accelerates the heart rate, however, it can produce extra heart beats (extra systoles) and cause palpitations (an annoying sensation of a pronounced or irregular heartbeat). Furthermore, in individuals who have periodic irregular heart beats (atrial fibrillation), this stimulant may increase the frequency of these episodes. Caffeine may also provoke heartburn, diarrhea, or constipation; aggravate ulcers in the stomach; and increase urination.

Some studies suggest that consumption of one to five cups of coffee daily may contribute to the development of permanent hypertension. Other reports indicate that caffeine does not cause sustained hypertension and that individuals develop a tolerance to caffeine; that is, the effect wears off.

In the past few decades, consumption of decaffeinated coffee has increased dramatically, particularly with the advent of decaffeinated beans,

Table 8. *Amounts of Caffeine in Some Common Foods and Beverages*

Source	Caffeine (mg)
Coffee, ³/₄ cup (6 fl oz/180 mL)	
Brewed, drip	103
Instant	57
Decaffeinated, brewed and instant	2
Espresso (single)	
Regular	100
Decaffeinated	5
Tea, ³/₄ cup (6 fl oz/180 mL)	
Black, brewed 3 minutes	40
Instant	30
Decaffeinated	1
Soft drinks, 1¹/₂ cups (12 fl oz/360 mL)	
Cola type, regular and diet	31 to 70
Noncola type	0 to 55
Chocolate	
Cocoa, dry powder, 1 tablespoon	10
Baking chocolate, 1 oz (30 g)	25
Chocolate milk, 1 cup (8 fl oz/250 mL)	10
Milk chocolate bar, 1¹/₂ oz (45 g)	10

Source: Bowes and Church's food values of portions commonly used, 17th ed. Lippincott-Raven Publishers, 1998. By permission.

which permit brewing and improve flavor to the point where one cannot tell the difference between regular and decaffeinated coffee. Perhaps one of five coffee drinkers uses the decaffeinated form to avoid any effects of caffeine. In the United States, decaffeinated coffee is routinely made available wherever regular coffee is served. Indeed, only decaffeinated coffee is served following dinner at many social gatherings and private parties. The demand for decaffeinated tea and cola drinks has also increased somewhat. Obviously, if one has several cups of coffee and also drinks tea and caffeinated soft drinks during the day, the amount of caffeine consumed can be considerable and result in undesirable side effects. Thus it is wise to keep track of your caffeinated drink consumption.

Although no strong evidence implicates caffeine as a cause of permanent hypertension, **it is reasonable for persons who already have hyper-**

tension to avoid repeated elevations of blood pressure, particularly if these increases are exacerbated by consumption of caffeinated drinks. For persons with hypertension who regularly consume considerable amounts of caffeine, it would be wise to check the effect of drinking a cup of regular coffee on blood pressure and heart rate. If elevations of blood pressure are pronounced (systolic or diastolic elevations of 5 to 10 mm Hg), or if the heart rate is markedly increased or irregularities occur, then it is recommended that consumption of caffeinated drinks be significantly reduced or replaced with consumption of decaffeinated drinks.

Many experts recommend that daily caffeine consumption be limited to about 200 milligrams (mg) per day (two cups of coffee, four cups of tea, or no more than two to four cans of caffeinated sodas) in patients with hypertension. In addition, caffeinated drinks should be avoided immediately before strenuous physical activities. Likewise, such drinks should be avoided for at least one hour before blood pressure is measured so that an accurate reading, uninfluenced by caffeine, can be obtained.

Although some have reported that excess coffee consumption may cause some elevation of "bad" cholesterol (LDL—low-density lipoprotein) and triglycerides in the blood, the evidence is not compelling. Any slight changes are probably of no importance. In fact, after tolerance to caffeine develops, caffeinated drinks have no effect on blood pressure or heart rate.

Finally, one study has reported that men consuming lots of tea, which contains antioxidants, have a reduced chance of heart attack (see Question 96). This interesting finding remains to be confirmed.

57. Is It Safe to Take Estrogen Before and After Menopause If You Have Hypertension?

Oral contraceptives ("the pill"), when initially introduced, contained relatively high concentrations of two female hormones, estrogen and progesterone. Such high hormone concentrations may possibly cause salt retention and an increased blood volume, as well as other changes that result in constriction of arterioles with elevation of blood pressure. The exact cause of the elevated blood pressure remains unclear, however. With the original oral contraceptives, 5% to 18% of the women taking these oral contraceptives would develop mild elevations of blood pressure. Fortunately, their blood pressures returned to normal after discontinuing the medication. The high doses of estrogens and progesterone in the original oral contraceptives were associated with blood clots and strokes. In men, high concentrations of estrogen can also increase the risk of cardiovascular disease such as heart attack and stroke.

Subsequently, the concentrations of estrogen and progesterone in "the pill" were considerably reduced. Today, oral contraceptives rarely increase blood pressure. Estrogens alone taken in very high dosages may increase blood pressure, although low dosages do not bring about hypertension and may actually reduce blood pressure. This situation is one in which more is not necessarily better.

Estrogens alone taken in very high dosages may increase blood pressure, although low dosages do not bring about hypertension and may actually reduce blood pressure.

The effectiveness of estrogen replacement therapy (ERT) in low dosage, administered as a pill or skin patch, is readily evident in two instances:

- In the treatment of osteoporosis
- In controlling menopausal symptoms such as hot flashes and vaginal dryness

A number of studies indicate that estrogens decrease the risk of heart disease.

The explanation for the lower risk of heart and blood vessel disease and stroke in premenopausal women compared to men of similar age probably depends on the fact that premenopausal women have lower blood pressures and lower levels of "bad" cholesterol (LDL—low-density lipoprotein) and higher levels of "good" cholesterol (HDL—high-density lipoprotein) than men. These favorable cholesterol levels are likely related to the high levels of estrogen in premenopausal women. After menopause, women lose these cardiovascular protective factors due to the marked reduction of estrogen in their circulation. As a result, their risk of cardiovascular disease is equal to or even greater than that in men of the same age. A three-year study of 875 postmenopausal women by the National Institutes of Health revealed that ERT decreased LDL by about 20% and increased HDL; blood pressure did not increase and there was no increase in the occurrence of cancers. Nevertheless, it is important to recognize that the incidence of cancer of the uterus may be doubled in postmenopausal women taking ERT as compared with postmenopausal women not using estrogen. Whether estrogen increases the incidence of breast cancer in postmenopausal women remains controversial.

In deciding who to treat with ERT, the physician and patient must weigh the value of the treatment against the possible risks. **As the small**

dosage of estrogen with or without progesterone does not increase blood pressure, there is no contraindication to its use because of the presence of hypertension. ERT is indicated in postmenopausal women who have a strong family history of cardiovascular disease and either elevated LDL and/or other potentially harmful fats (such as triglycerides) or low HDL, unless there is a strong reason against its use. However, even a low concentration of estrogen is not given to men to protect them from cardiovascular disease, because it causes impotence and breast enlargement. If there is a family history of osteoporosis or if osteoporosis is evident by bone density studies, then ERT is indicated in combination with calcium and vitamin D supplements; such patients should also undertake adequate weight-bearing exercise with or without one of the new nonhormonal drugs (Fosamax) that enhance calcium deposition in bones.

To protect patients from the possibility of developing uterine cancer while on ERT, progesterone should be added to the treatment. This hormone will help to counteract the stimulatory effect of estrogen on the lining of the uterus and thus reduce the chance of uterine cancer. It is noteworthy that the combination of estrogen and progesterone can slightly increase the chance of blood clots and gallbladder disease. Of course, if a hysterectomy has been performed previously, then progesterone need not be added. Finally, ERT is not recommended in patients who have had breast cancer or who have a family history of breast cancer.

A newly developed estrogen-like drug (Evista) for osteoporosis may eventually be used in place of estrogen, as it seems as effective for osteoporosis as estrogen but does not appear to increase the risk of uterine or breast cancer. Unfortunately, Evista does not seem to have the same beneficial effect on cardiovascular disease that estrogen has.

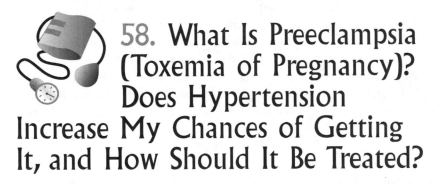

58. What Is Preeclampsia (Toxemia of Pregnancy)? Does Hypertension Increase My Chances of Getting It, and How Should It Be Treated?

Preeclampsia occurs in approximately 3% of all pregnancies, most often during the first pregnancy. It is usually characterized by hypertension, retention of water and salt (manifested by swelling of the ankles, face, and hands, plus weight gain), and increased protein in the urine in the third trimester of pregnancy. This condition was originally called toxemia of pregnancy, because it was thought to result from a toxin that appeared in the circulation after the twentieth week of pregnancy. Today, however, physicians consider the cause of the condition to be a mystery.

Normally diastolic blood pressure decreases 5 to 10 mm Hg, with little change in systolic pressure, during the first and second trimesters; it then returns to its initial level in the third trimester. Preeclampsia occurs most frequently in the following women:

- Young women (in their teens) or women older than 40 years of age during their first pregnancy
- Women with a family history of preeclampsia
- Women carrying multiple fetuses
- African American women
- Women with preexisting hypertension, diabetes, kidney disease, or obesity
- Women who have had preeclampsia in a former pregnancy

Recognizing preeclampsia and treating it appropriately are extremely important to prevent the development of a very serious condition known as eclampsia. The latter condition occurs in about 1 in 1500 pregnancies and is associated with pronounced hypertension, severe headaches, visual disturbances, abdominal pains, seizures, unconsciousness, and even death of mother and fetus.

The presence of high blood pressure before pregnancy should not deter you from becoming pregnant, as your pregnancy may be completely normal (see Question 59). Nevertheless, because the presence of hypertension increases the risk for preeclampsia, blood pressure should be carefully monitored in hypertensive women with appropriate medication during pregnancy. Aldomet has been used successfully for many years and has proved safe for both mother and fetus. Beta blockers and the vasodilator, Apresoline, also appear effective and safe, and diuretics ("water pills") may occasionally be indicated. Other antihypertensive medications should usually be discontinued and avoided in pregnancy, especially the ACE inhibitors and angiotensin II receptor blockers, because they may retard growth of the fetus and cause birth defects and even death of the fetus. In patients with preeclampsia, the drugs mentioned above (with the exception of diuretics) can be used, bed rest is sometimes indicated (to lower blood pressure and to improve blood flow to the fetus), and hospitalization may be required. Early delivery by cesarean section will rapidly

The presence of high blood pressure before pregnancy should not deter you from becoming pregnant, as your pregnancy may be completely normal.

resolve the symptoms and signs of severe preeclampsia, prevent the development of eclampsia, and return the blood pressure to the level it was before the onset of pregnancy.

It should be emphasized that women with hypertension or other risks for preeclampsia who are planning to become pregnant should be followed closely by physicians who have expertise in managing hypertension.

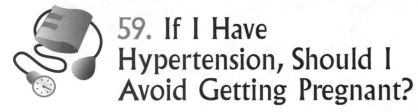

59. If I Have Hypertension, Should I Avoid Getting Pregnant?

Hypertensive women do not necessarily have to avoid pregnancy. It is a good sign if you have had a previous uncomplicated pregnancy. If your hypertension is not severe, you have a good chance of carrying a pregnancy to term without a problem. You should, however, be under the supervision of an obstetrician from the very outset of the pregnancy. If you are taking an ACE inhibitor or an angiotensin II receptor blocker (see Question 58) for your hypertension, you should stop using the medication before you become pregnant or as soon as you know you are pregnant, because these drugs may cause fetal damage or mortality. If you have severe hypertension (blood pressure of more than 180/110 mm Hg), you should consult your physician and an obstetrician before becoming pregnant.

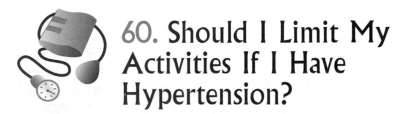

60. Should I Limit My Activities If I Have Hypertension?

You should limit your activities only if you have already developed complications from hypertension, such as heart disease, kidney disease, or stroke. In general, aerobic exercise (running, walking, jogging, swimming, and so on) is beneficial for hypertension, because it may lower blood pressure, improve cardiovascular fitness, and help in reducing excess weight. For patients with uncomplicated hypertension, there is no benefit from restricting activities or cutting back on your workload. If complications such as heart disease, kidney disease, or stroke have already occurred, your physician will advise you about limiting your activities. Typically, the physician may recommend a supervised, graded exercise program.

Before embarking on any exercise program, most physicians believe that it is prudent for most individuals older than 45 years to obtain a stress test. Such a test records the electrical activity of your heart while you are exercising on a treadmill. This information is very helpful in determining any abnormalities of the blood supply to the heart, which might make strenuous exercise inadvisable.

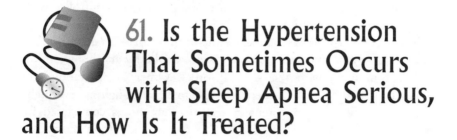

61. Is the Hypertension That Sometimes Occurs with Sleep Apnea Serious, and How Is It Treated?

Sleep apnea is a periodic cessation of breathing during sleep (see Question 38). It usually lasts anywhere from 20 seconds to 3 minutes and may occur from 10 to 15 times per hour. This sleep disorder affects 2% to 4% of middle-aged women and men. Two types of sleep apnea are recognized: that caused by airway obstruction in the pharyngeal area, and that caused by decreased activity of the nerve impulses that drive the respiratory muscles.

Airway obstruction in the pharyngeal area (back of the mouth and upper airway tube) may result from anatomical disturbances in the back of the mouth or tongue with "pharyngeal crowding." Obesity often contributes to the problem, and alcohol consumption can aggravate it. Loud snoring is extremely common, often associated with cessation of breathing, choking or gasping, and is frequently witnessed by the bed partner or someone else. Chronic sleepiness during the day, intellectual deterioration, personality changes, behavioral disorders, memory loss, and impotence may occur. Furthermore, these episodes of apnea may be accompanied by slowing or speeding up of the heart rate, development of hypertension, stroke, heart attack, and premature death.

Episodes of obstructive sleep apnea may be accompanied by slowing or speeding up of the heart rate, development of hypertension, stroke, heart attack, and premature death.

The diagnosis of this type of sleep apnea can be confirmed by an overnight sleep study with appropriate recordings to determine brain waves, muscle activity, and oxygen deficiency. Treatment consists of weight reduction (if indicated), avoidance of alcohol, avoidance of sleeping in the supine position (on the back), use of oral devices to keep the airway open at night, and use of a pressure apparatus to deliver air continuously to the patient at night. Occasionally, surgical procedures to ameliorate the obstructed airflow may be necessary. If the episodes of hypertension are modest and occur only in conjunction with the apnea, antihypertensive medication is probably not indicated. On the other hand, if the patient already has hypertension and a marked rise in blood pressure occurs during apnea, then it is important that blood pressure be controlled with antihypertensive medication.

The second type of sleep apnea results from a *decreased activity of the nerve impulses that drive the respiratory muscles.* Obesity and hypertension are less prominent with this sleep disorder. Other manifestations are similar to patients with obstructive sleep apnea, although an overnight sleep study will reveal recurrent apneas that are not accompanied by respiratory effort. In individuals with this condition, carbon dioxide in the blood tends to progressively increase during the night. Some patients benefit from continuous air delivery with a pressure apparatus and from delivery of oxygen.

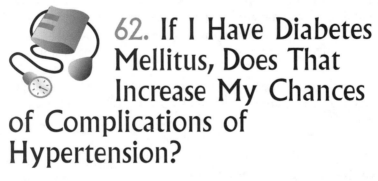

62. If I Have Diabetes Mellitus, Does That Increase My Chances of Complications of Hypertension?

Diabetes mellitus is definitely linked to greater risk of hypertension complications. **The combination of diabetes and hypertension is a bad one because either condition can lead to premature heart attacks, strokes, and kidney failure, but when the two conditions occur together, the outlook is even worse** (see Question 43). We recommend that diabetic/hypertensive patients receive aggressive treatment for both conditions. In these patients, the goal of treatment for hypertension should be to reduce blood pressure to less than 130/85 mm Hg. Close control of the blood sugar is also helpful in this situation.

63. Will Antihypertensive Drugs Interfere with My Physical or Mental Activity and be a Danger to My Health?

Very rarely will antihypertensive drugs interfere with mental function or physical activity, and they should never be a danger to your health, when properly administered. Remember, it is always better to treat hypertension than to leave it untreated. Nevertheless, some medications should not be used in patients who require maximal physical performance or who compete in amateur and professional athletic events. Furthermore, some antihypertensive agents may impair mental alertness, which could pose a hazard when driving an automobile or working with dangerous machinery.

Beta blockers slow the heart rate, can slightly decrease exercise tolerance, and may rarely cause fatigue; they would, therefore, be a poor choice for anyone engaged in strenuous sports. These drugs may also cause bronchospasm in some patients, especially those with asthma, which could further compromise exercise enjoyment and athletic performance. Depression has occasionally been observed with some beta blockers (those that reach the brain). In a small percentage of men, such agents may lead to impotence and loss of sex desire and further aggravate depression. The long-acting diuretics may also cause impotence in a small percentage of men (see Question 66).

Beta blockers slow the heart rate, can slightly decrease exercise tolerance, and may rarely cause fatigue; they would, therefore, be a poor choice for anyone engaged in strenuous sports.

If beta blockers are discontinued, the dosage should be decreased gradually over a number of days in patients with evidence of coronary artery disease. The gradual weaning is necessary to avoid any risk of heart attack.

Clonidine (Catapres) acts on the central nervous system and lowers blood pressure by decreasing the activity of the sympathetic nervous system, thereby permitting arterioles to dilate and blood pressure to decrease. In large doses, it can induce extreme fatigue, drowsiness, and sedation. Impaired thinking, psychological problems, and depression have been observed, and impotence may occur. Weakness and unsteadiness affect approximately 6% of patients. Certainly this drug should not be given to patients requiring alertness, normal reflex reaction time, and skillful coordination. Another concern with patients consuming sizable doses of clonidine is that this medication should never be stopped abruptly, as sudden termination may result in a very marked and potentially dangerous elevation of blood pressure.

Any antihypertensive drug can potentially lower blood pressure excessively and cause a feeling of faintness and unsteadiness, which could result in loss of consciousness and a fall with possible serious injury. Patients vary considerably in their blood pressure response to the various antihypertensive medications. Therefore, it is reasonable and prudent to start with relatively low doses of these drugs and to check the blood pressures of patients in both seated and standing positions. If a marked decrease of the blood pressure occurs when the patient stands up—a condition sometimes associated with faintness—then a smaller dose of the medication is indicated. **In a small percentage of patients, the alpha$_1$-blocking drugs (mainly Minipress) are particularly likely to cause a pronounced drop in blood pressure when standing within a short time after the first dose is taken.** For this reason, the first dose should be taken at bedtime rather than during the day, as having a recumbent position in bed will prevent the loss of consciousness that might occur in the standing position. Fortunately, after this possible first-dose effect, alpha$_1$ blockers can be used without fear of subsequent hypotensive episodes.

In general, when low to moderate doses of antihypertensive drugs are used, or when combinations of low or moderate doses of such drugs are used to control blood pressure, bothersome side effects are relatively few.

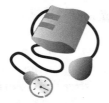

64. What Is a Hypertensive Emergency?

In a hypertensive emergency, high blood pressure is leading to damage in the target organs (heart, brain, kidneys), which can be prevented or minimized by aggressive treatment of the high blood pressure.

In a hypertensive emergency, high blood pressure is leading to damage in the target organs (heart, brain, kidneys), which can be prevented or minimized by aggressive treatment of the high blood pressure, sometimes with medications given by injection into a vein. Common hypertensive emergencies include heart failure with fluid in the lungs, signs of impending stroke, and evidence of kidney failure, as determined by urinalysis and blood tests. The typical hypertensive emergency is "hypertensive encephalopathy," a condition in which the brain swells because of the very high blood pressure and leads to severe headache, intermittent blindness, nausea, vomiting, and confusion.

The goal of treatment is to reduce blood pressure to nearly normal levels within three to four hours by giving blood-pressure-lowering medications by injection. **Hypertensive emergencies should not occur if high blood pressure is treated appropriately and effectively.** In fact, hypertensive encephalopathy has been seen only rarely since effective treatment of hypertension became available. When it does occur, it usually affects patients who have not had their hypertension treated or who have discontinued treatment.

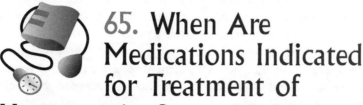

65. When Are Medications Indicated for Treatment of Hypertension?

Stroke, heart attack, heart and kidney failure, and hardening of the arteries all occur least frequently when blood pressures remain at 135/85 mm Hg or less. Establishing an accurate, average blood pressure level is therefore essential before starting treatment. It is important to determine whether elevated blood pressures obtained in the doctor's office might be due to anxiety ("white-coat hypertension"). In this endeavor, having the patient, a family member, or friend record the blood pressure at home can be very helpful in determining a truly accurate pressure (see Questions 14, 19). When taking blood pressure measurements, the patient should be in a seated position and relaxed in a quiet environment for at least five minutes before the pressure is recorded, and the blood pressure cuff should be the right size and placed at about the level of the sternum (breast bone). Cigarette smoking, consumption of drinks containing caffeine, and exercise should be avoided for approximately one hour before the blood pressure is measured. If blood pressures are only slightly elevated, lifestyle changes (such as reducing excess weight, limiting salt and alcohol intake, getting adequate exercise, and consuming a potassium-rich, low-fat diet) may reduce pressures into a normal range. Although it is doubtful that cigarette smoking contributes to the development of hypertension, cessation of smoking is still extremely important—there is no more serious health risk for heart and blood vessel disease, cancer, obstructive lung disease, and emphysema. Furthermore, smoking enhances a person's risk of developing the complications of hypertension (see Question 51).

If elevations of blood pressure (more than 140/90 mm Hg) persist despite lifestyle changes for three to six months, antihypertensive medication should be started. It is noteworthy that an elevated systolic blood pressure poses more of a risk for complications of hypertension than diastolic pressure elevations do (see Question 20). Therefore, even if only systolic pressures are elevated, treatment to normalize the pressure is indicated. With pressures of 160/100 mm Hg or greater, lifestyle changes and antihypertensive medications should be started immediately. Even if pressures are only mildly or moderately elevated, aggressive treatment with drugs and diet to lower blood pressure should be instituted if the patient has any evidence of heart, kidney, brain, or vascular disease. Only very rarely is hospitalization required to initiate very aggressive treatment (for example, when hypertension is very severe and/or accompanied by acute damage to the brain, heart, kidneys, and blood vessels).

If elevations of blood pressure (more than 140/90 mm Hg) persist despite lifestyle changes for three to six months, antihypertensive medication should be started.

66. What Are the Various Drugs Available for Treating Hypertension? How Do They Work and What Are Their Side Effects? Are Generic Medications As Good As Brand-Name Drugs?

Although the choice of antihypertensive drugs depends somewhat on age, gender, race, accompanying diseases, and medical history, the main objective of treatment is to normalize blood pressure and to prevent and/or reduce damage to the brain, heart, kidneys, and blood vessels. The final decision regarding the choice of medications should always be left to the attending physician, who knows the patient best. Appropriate lifestyle changes should always be initiated; they will usually have a beneficial effect on the patient's health as well as lower blood pressure and often reduce the amount of medication needed for blood pressure control.

Currently, more than 80 antihypertensive medications are commercially available in the United States. Most are single drugs, though some consist of combinations of two drugs. The commonly used oral antihypertensive medications (those taken by mouth) include diuretics, beta blockers, ACE inhibitors, angiotensin II (A II) receptor blockers, calcium-channel blockers, and alpha₁ blockers. Combinations of a diuretic with a potassium-conserving agent, a beta blocker, an ACE inhibitor, or an A II receptor blocker are also popular therapeutic options. Less commonly used antihypertensives include agents that lower blood pressure by depressing sympathetic nerve activity, thereby dilating arterioles. Table 9 lists most of the antihypertensives available in the United States and their mechanisms of action.

> *The commonly used oral antihypertensive medications include diuretics, beta blockers, ACE inhibitors, angiotensin II receptor blockers, calcium-channel blockers, and alpha₁ blockers.*

Combinations may be more convenient when the patient must take a large number of pills each day. Nevertheless, some physicians prefer to determine how individual drugs affect the patient before using them in combination, as one of the drugs used as single-agent therapy may adequately control the blood pressure. Furthermore, if undesirable side effects occur, it is often not possible to tell which drug in a combination is responsible. However, the trend now is to start with combination tablets. Combination drugs may be less expensive than two drugs purchased individually.

Long-acting diuretics (thiazides)—also known as "water pills"—have a duration of action of about 24 hours. They are highly effective, safe drugs with which to initiate treatment of hypertension. Their action on the kidney tubules eliminates salt and water and causes arteries to relax, thereby reducing blood pressure. Dietary salt should be limited when these agents are prescribed, because limiting salt consumption enhances the antihypertensive effect and may reduce the amount of diuretic required to reduce blood pressure. African Americans, the elderly, and obese individuals are often salt-sensitive; consequently, diuretics are particularly effective in these individuals.

Increased urination occurs when long-acting diuretics are initially taken, but is usually not a problem unless the patient has significant prostatic obstruction. Although these drugs are associated with few side effects, a small percentage of males may experience impotence with them. Occasionally, the level of potassium in the blood decreases significantly, which may alter the rhythm of the heart. The lower doses of diuretics now used routinely ensure that the problem of low blood potassium is a rare one. In addition, low-potassium problems can be prevented by prescribing a potassium-conserving agent (a weak diuretic) combined with the

Table 9. *Brand Names of Some Antihypertensive Drugs Commonly Used in the United States*

Diuretics
(cause excretion of salt and water, and dilate blood vessels)

Long-acting thiazide diuretics (act on distal tubule in kidneys)
- Diucardin
- Diuril
- Enduron
- Esidrix
- Hydrochlorothiazide
- HydroDiuril
- Hygroton
- Lozol
- Mykrox
- Naqua
- Naturetin
- Oretic
- Renese
- Thalitone
- Zaroxolyn

Short-acting diuretics (act on loop tubule in kidneys)
- Bumex
- Demadex (long-acting)
- Edecrin
- Lasix

Potassium-sparing diuretics (weak diuretics cause kidneys to retain potassium)
- Aldactone
- Dyrenium
- Midamor

Beta Blockers
(diminish effect of norepinephrine and epinephrine on heart and blood vessels)

- Blocadren
- Cartrol
- Corgard
- Inderal, Inderal LA
- Kerlone
- Levatol
- Lopressor (metoprolol)
- Sectral
- Tenormin
- Toprol-XL (metoprolol)
- Visken
- Zebeta

Table 9. *Continued*

ACE Inhibitors (prevent production of angiotensin II)	• Accupril • Altace • Capoten • Lotensin • Mavik • Monopril • Prinivil • Univasc • Vasotec • Zestril
Angiotensin II Blockers (block the effect of angiotensin II on receptors of this hormone in blood vessels and the adrenal gland)	• Atacand • Avapro • Cozaar • Diovan • Teveten
Calcium-Channel Blockers (long-acting) (block entry of calcium into heart or blood vessel cells)	*Nondihydropyridines* (cause vasodilation and slow electrical conduction of the heart) • Calan SR • Cardizem CD, Cardizem SR • Covera HS • Dilacor XR • Isoptin SR • Tiazac • Verelan *Dihydropyridines* (cause only dilation of arteries and no effect on heart) • Adalat CC • Cardene XL • DynaCirc • Norvasc • Plendil • Procardia XL • Sular
Alpha$_1$ Blockers (diminish the constricting action of norepinephrine and epinephrine on blood vessels)	• Cardura (long-acting) • Hytrin (long-acting) • Minipress (short-acting)

(Continued)

Table 9. *Continued*

Alpha₂ Agonists (cause depression of the sympathetic nervous system that results in vasodilation)	• Aldomet • Catapres • Tenex • Wytensin
Combination Drugs	*Alpha₁ and beta blocker* (diminishes effect of epinephrine and norepinephrine on alpha₁ and beta receptors) • Coreg • Normodyne • Trandate

Alpha₁ and beta blocker (diminishes effect of epinephrine and norepinephrine on alpha₁ and beta receptors)
• Coreg
• Normodyne
• Trandate

Diuretic and beta blocker (increases elimination of salt and water and diminishes effect of norepinephrine and epinephrine on beta receptors)
• Corzide
• Inderide LA (long-acting)
• Lopressor HCT (hydrochlorothiazide)
• Tenoretic
• Timolide
• Ziac

Diuretic and ACE inhibitor (increases elimination of salt and water and inhibits formation of angiotensin, which can increase blood pressure, thereby preventing hypertension)
• Capozide
• Lotensin HCT
• Prinzide
• Vaseretic
• Zestoretic

Diuretic and angiotensin receptor antagonist (increases elimination of salt and water and prevents action of angiotensin on receptors, thereby reducing blood pressure)
• Avalide
• Diovan HCT (hydrochlorothiazide)
• Hyzaar

Potassium-sparing and thiazide diuretic (increases elimination of salt and water but prevents elimination of potassium)
• Aldactazide
• Dyazide

Table 9. *Continued*

Combination Drugs *(Cont.)*	• Maxzide • Moduretic *Calcium antagonist and ACE inhibitor* (inhibits calcium from causing constriction of arteries and inhibits the formation of angiotensin, thereby reducing blood pressure) • Lexxel • Lotrel • Tarka • Teczem
Adrenergic Depleters (diminish norepinephrine in sympathetic nerves which results in vasodilation)	• Hylorel • Ismelin • Reserpine
Vasodilators (cause vasodilation by directly causing muscles in the vessels to relax)	• Apresazide (a combination of Apresoline plus hydrochlorothiazide) • Apresoline • Loniten

thiazide, if the thiazide causes a significant decrease of potassium in the blood. Gout may be precipitated by use of diuretics, so these drugs should be used cautiously if the patient has a history of gout.

Loop diuretics affect a different part of the kidney tubule than that targeted by long-acting diuretics. In addition, they are more potent and have a more rapid onset of action than thiazides. These short-acting (four to six hours) drugs are indicated if the patient has severely impaired kidney function or heart failure, because they are more effective in eliminating salt and water than the long-acting diuretics are. Loop diuretics must be taken twice daily, and they do not decrease the blood pressure as effectively as the thiazides. Because impaired kidney function can lead to potassium retention, drugs that decrease potassium excretion are contra-indicated in patients with poor kidney function.

Beta blockers are antihypertensive agents that block two hormones—norepinephrine (released from the sympathetic nervous system) and epi-nephrine (released from adrenal gland)—from reaching their receptors in the heart. In this way, these blockers reduce heart rate and its pumping action, and some diminish resistance (constriction) in arterioles. In addi-tion, beta blockers suppress production of renin in the kidney, thereby preventing the formation of angiotensin II (a powerful constrictor of arteries). As a result of all these actions, the blood pressure decreases.

Beta blockers provide another benefit by reducing the work of the heart and its oxygen requirement in patients who have angina (pain or a pressure sensation in the chest due to a deficient oxygen supply to the heart). Such drugs can help control rapid and irregular heart rhythm, and they have been shown to reduce the chance of a second heart attack. In addition, beta blockers may be beneficial in treating heart failure.

Beta blockers must be administered cautiously, however, as sometimes they may worsen heart failure and may impair electrical conduction in the heart. Because blocking beta receptors in the lung can cause bronchial constriction, these drugs may precipitate or aggravate asthmatic attacks. They can also be associated with fatigue, decreased exercise tolerance, and cold hands; some users may experience impotence and decreased sexual drive. Luckily, most individuals experience few of these side effects. A slight increase in blood fats (triglycerides) and a decrease in "good" cholesterol (HDL) may occur, but are usually not very significant. In patients receiving insulin, beta blockers may mask the symptoms of low blood sugar. Some beta blockers mainly affect the heart, whereas others have a more generalized effect and reach the brain and may cause depression.

ACE (angiotensin-converting enzyme) inhibitors restrain the formation of angiotensin II, a powerful constrictor of arteries, which may also retain salt and water. These drugs also permit a buildup of bradykinin, a substance that causes dilation of blood vessels. The end result—lower blood pressure. ACE inhibitors are not only effective as antihypertensive drugs, but also valuable in treating heart failure, especially when the disease is caused by hypertension, and in slowing the progression of kidney failure in diabetics. With severe kidney failure, however, ACE inhibitors may aggravate the failure and cause retention of potassium. In general, physicians avoid potassium-sparing drugs and potassium supplementation in patients taking ACE inhibitors.

Approximately 10% to 20% of all people who take these drugs develop a dry, hacking cough, which may require its discontinuance. They may also cause a skin rash or diminish one's sense of taste; very rarely an acute allergic reaction is accompanied by swelling of the tongue and face. ACE inhibitors should not be used during pregnancy or if pregnancy is anticipated, because they may cause serious birth defects and fetal death.

Angiotensin II receptor blockers inhibit the effects of angiotensin II, thereby preventing constriction of blood vessels and retention of salt and water; as a consequence, blood pressure is lowered. Unlike ACE inhibitors, these drugs do not cause an increase in bradykinin or produce a dry cough. Allergic reactions and side effects are very rare. Like ACE inhibitors, angiotensin II inhibitors should be avoided during pregnancy or if pregnancy is planned. If potassium is elevated in the blood, these drugs should be avoided.

Calcium antagonists (calcium-channel blockers) consist of two types:

- The dihydropyridines, which cause blood vessels to dilate
- The nondihydropyridines, which cause blood vessel dilation but also slow down electrical conduction in the heart

Both types of drugs exert their effects by blocking calcium channels and thus diminishing access of calcium to the smooth muscles of the blood vessels. In addition, the nondihydropyridines diminish access of calcium to the muscles of the heart. Blood pressure is lowered by the vasodilation, which also increases blood supply to the heart and can be helpful in treating patients with angina (pain or a pressure sensation in the chest from diminished blood and oxygen to the heart). Likewise, calcium antagonists may benefit individuals with narrowed arteries in the legs, and they are particularly effective in elderly patients and individuals with systolic hypertension. Because they slow electrical conduction in the heart, the nondihydropyridines can be effective in the treatment of some heart irregularities, but they should not be used when electrical conduction in the heart is impaired, heart failure is present, or the patient is already taking beta blockers. Some nondihydropyridine calcium antagonists may be indicated in patients following a heart attack, if beta blockers cannot be used.

Side effects of calcium antagonists include constipation (only nondihydropyridines), swelling of the lower legs and feet, headaches, swollen gums, rash, and rapid heart beat (only dihydropyridines). Consumption of grapefruit juice can impair the liver's ability to eliminate some of these drugs, so this juice should not be consumed two hours before or two hours after taking calcium antagonists, as their accumulation in the body may become toxic.

About six years ago, concern was raised regarding the safety of short-acting dihydropyridines. Some reports indicated that the rapid and pronounced drop in blood pressure caused by these drugs might result in a stroke or heart attack in persons with heart disease. Subsequently, long-acting dihydropyridines have been developed and replaced the short-acting versions in the treatment of hypertension. The long-acting drugs produce a slow decline in blood pressure that persists for about 24 hours and is not hazardous to patients, even in the presence of heart disease.

Alpha₁ blockers inhibit the effect of norepinephrine, a hormone that is released from the sympathetic nerves. Normally norepinephrine constricts arteries; however, blocking its action causes dilation of arteries and thus reduces blood pressure. Alpha₁ blockers may improve urinary flow in men with partial urinary obstruction due to an enlarged prostate. In addition, they may increase "good" cholesterol (HDL) in blood and modestly lower total cholesterol and triglycerides. Rarely, the first dose may cause a pronounced drop in blood pressure with dizziness or fainting on standing. This effect is usually not a problem if the first dose is taken at bedtime, when the patient is recumbent, or if a small dose is given initially. Other potential side effects include headaches, nasal congestion, dry mouth, and rarely urinary incontinence in women.

Alpha$_2$ agonists exert their effects in the brain and diminish the activity of the sympathetic nerves to the arteries and heart. As a result, the smooth muscles in the arteries relax and the arteries dilate. Heart rate does not increase, however, and the blood pressure is reduced. These drugs are not used very often because of their potential side effects—sedation, drowsiness, decreased alertness, and fatigue—which may significantly disrupt mental and physical performance. Nevertheless, they may be beneficial in patients experiencing panic attacks or symptoms of withdrawal from alcohol or drug addiction.

The alpha$_2$ agonist Catapres can be applied to the skin in a patch, which is effective for one week and appears to cause fewer side effects than when taken as a pill. The "dry mouth" effect produced by some of these drugs can be particularly annoying. In addition, these antihypertensive agents may cause impotence and mental depression. Aldomet is a popular option in patients who are pregnant because of its safety and efficacy.

Stopping the use of some alpha$_2$ agonists abruptly may cause the blood pressure to increase rapidly to very high levels—high enough to cause a stroke. Therefore, gradual discontinuance of those drugs and physician consultation are important when weaning the patient away from them.

Combinations of alpha$_1$ and beta blockers are available as Normodyne, Trandate, and Coreg. These combination drugs lower blood pressure by decreasing constriction of arteries (due to alpha blockade) but have little effect on the pumping action of the heart (from beta blockade). In high concentration, Coreg exhibits a calcium-channel-blocking action. It may also neutralize toxic substances known as free radicals, thereby preventing damage to the lining of blood vessels. (Free radicals are harmful oxidation products in the body, which can be destroyed by antioxidants.)

On rare occasions, the combination therapies may cause a pronounced drop in blood pressure on standing, an effect that is more likely to occur at initiation of treatment and with large doses. These drugs may also cause failure to ejaculate, itching of the scalp, asthmatic-like breathing, skin eruptions, and rarely severe liver damage.

Adrenergic depleters cause depletion in sympathetic nerves of norepinephrine (the hormone released from these nerves). By so doing, they cause dilation of arteries and a decrease in blood pressure. Today these drugs are rarely used because of their side effects (reserpine may cause gastric ulceration and serious mental depression; Ismelin and Hylorel can cause a pronounced drop in blood pressure on standing, ejaculation failure, fluid retention, and diarrhea). Indeed, many more acceptable drugs for the treatment of hypertension are available.

Vasodilators act directly on the muscles in the walls of arteries, causing them to dilate and thereby reducing blood pressure. These powerful dilators of the arteries are often used in patients who do not respond to other antihypertensive medications.

Loniten is more potent than Apresoline and is especially valuable in the therapy of severe hypertension accompanied by impairment of kidney function. Loniten can lead to retention of salt and water, so this agent is frequently used in combination with diuretics (water pills). Apresoline usually causes rapid heart rate, which may aggravate pain or a pressure sensation in the chest (angina); therefore beta blockers are often employed along with this drug to slow the heart rate and prevent the angina. Other potential side effects include flushing and headaches. Apresoline can also rarely cause a connective tissue disease similar to lupus (which usually subsides on discontinuation of the drug), and Loniten causes hair growth over the entire body in about 80% of patients, including women.

Some antihypertensive drugs are available only as brand-name version, because the pharmaceutical company that originally develops the drug has 17 years before its patent rights expire and hence generic versions can be marketed. **The generic drugs that are available are identical in activity and side effects to their brand-name predecessors.** You can be sure they have been carefully tested and evaluated by the Food and Drug Administration. Thus there is no reason to avoid using the cheaper generic-named antihypertensive medications when they are available.

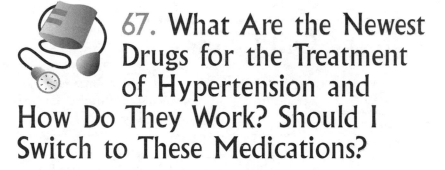

67. What Are the Newest Drugs for the Treatment of Hypertension and How Do They Work? Should I Switch to These Medications?

A new class of drugs, vasopeptidase inhibitors (VPIs), may soon be available for treatment of hypertension. These drugs possess a dual beneficial action:

- They are ACE inhibitors.
- They inhibit the breakdown of hormones known as natriuretic peptides, which cause dilation of arterioles and increase salt and water elimination.

These actions can very effectively reduce blood pressure.

A new class of drugs, vasopeptidase inhibitors, may soon be available for treatment of hypertension.

One VPI, Vanlev (its generic name is omapatrilat), may become commercially available in 2001. Clinical studies indicate that it has a pronounced and greater effect on reducing systolic blood pressure than on reducing diastolic blood pressure, which would make it especially desirable for treating patients with only systolic hypertension. Many other VPIs are in the drug development pipeline as well. Their commercialization may provide a valuable and significant advancement in the management of hypertension, providing that no serious side effects are encountered; further evaluation is needed.

"Newer" does not necessarily mean "better" when it comes to antihypertensive medications. Some older drugs have excellent track records for successfully controlling blood pressure and preventing complications of hypertension, cause few if any side effects, and are relatively inexpensive. **If your blood pressure is under good control and you are experiencing no side effects, you should continue with your current medication.** Any decision to change medication should be made in consultation with your physician.

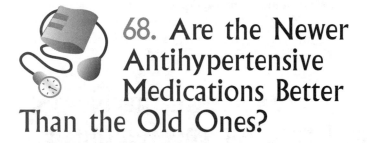

68. Are the Newer Antihypertensive Medications Better Than the Old Ones?

Newer medications have not demonstrated any convincing superiority relative to older antihypertensive drugs in lowering blood pressure.

Clinical trials comparing newer medications to the older ones have not demonstrated any convincing superiority for the newer drugs in lowering blood pressure. In general, the newcomers appear no more effective in reducing blood pressure than the older ones, nor are they more effective in reducing complications of hypertension. The exception is the ACE inhibitor drug class, which has shown superior benefits in diabetic patients who have protein (albumin) in the urine and in patients with heart failure. ACE inhibitors can improve blood flow in the kidneys, reduce protein in the urine, and prevent progression of kidney disease (better than other antihypertensive drugs, in the latter case). They also reduce the workload on a failing heart. On the other hand, the beta blockers (an older class of antihypertensive drugs) are the most effective in preventing recurrent heart attacks in hypertensive patients as well as in patients who have normal blood pressure.

69. What Medications Will My Doctor Prescribe for My Hypertension? When Are Certain Drugs Indicated or When Should They Be Avoided (Contraindicated)?

Most specialists who treat hypertension agree with the guidelines recently proposed by the Joint National Committee on Prevention, Detection, Evaluation, and Treatment of High Blood Pressure (JNC VI report). This committee, which meets periodically as part of the National High Blood Pressure Education Program, is composed of approximately 45 prestigious organizations that have interest and expertise in the management of hypertension. The recommendations of this committee are very logical and reasonable, because they are based on years of experience with most of the antihypertensive drugs.

"Newer" does not necessarily mean "better" with antihypertensives. It should be appreciated that diuretics and beta blockers have the longest track record in treating hypertension, and their ability to decrease complications and mortality from hypertension has been established by many carefully controlled studies. A long-acting thiazide diuretic (water pill) or a beta blocker may be recommended by your physician as initial therapy, if no good medical reasons exist not to use these drugs. This recommendation holds true for the vast majority of patients with mild to moderately severe hypertension—that is, with blood pressures less than 180/110 mm Hg. The presence of risk factors (such as diabetes, smoking,

Diuretics and beta blockers have the longest track record in treating hypertension, and their ability to decrease complications and mortality from hypertension has been established by many carefully controlled studies.

obesity, high blood cholesterol, or a family history of a heart attack or stroke at a relatively young age) or evidence of pathologic changes caused by hypertension (such as heart disease, stroke, kidney function impairment, or damage to arteries of the eyes or legs) necessitates the use of more aggressive treatment. Your physician will usually select a combination of drugs that most effectively treats your hypertension and risk factors.

In general, when nonpharmacological measures (for example, excess weight loss, limitation of salt and alcohol consumption, and increasing exercise) do not normalize the blood pressure, antihypertensive drugs should be started with the objective of lowering blood pressure to an optimal level of about 130/80 mm Hg or less. In those individuals requiring antihypertensive medication, one drug adequately controls high blood pressure in almost 50% of patients with stage 1 or stage 2 hypertension. With severe (stage 3) hypertension (blood pressures equal to or greater than 180/110 mm Hg), two antihypertensive drugs will be sufficient to normalize blood pressure in approximately 80% of hypertensives. Additional medication will be required for individuals who prove more resistant to treatment. The ways in which oral antihypertensive drugs work and their side effects were discussed in Question 66. Here we make some general comments about the use of these medications, then describe indications for specific drugs for patients with hypertension complicated by a variety of other medical conditions.

A long-acting thiazide (water pill) is often recommended as initial therapy in individuals with essential hypertension (that is, patients in whom all known causes of secondary hypertension have been eliminated) **who have no significant impairment of kidney function and no history of gout (joint inflammation).** Because diuretics can cause loss of potassium in the urine, which might lead to a serious irregularity of the heart rhythm, some physicians prefer to use a small to moderate dose of a potassium-sparing diuretic and periodically check the effect of this drug on the serum concentration of potassium. The rare occurrence of impotence may require discontinuance in some men. Even small doses of thiazide diuretics will normalize blood pressure in approximately 50% of individuals, and these agents are the least expensive of all antihypertensive drugs. The diuretics are particularly effective in older adults (especially in those with only systolic hypertension) and in African Americans and other individuals with salt-sensitive hypertension (that is, in individuals who retain salt).

Beta blockers may also be used as initial treatment in hypertension. They are contraindicated or should be used cautiously if the patient has a history of asthma or chronic lung disease that could be aggravated by the constriction of air passages in the lungs—an effect sometimes linked to these drugs. Furthermore, beta blockers should not be given to patients with impairment of the electrical conduction system in the heart, as they could further slow the conduction system and the heart rate.

Originally concern was raised that these drugs might worsen heart failure; however, they have been shown to be of value in treating some forms of heart failure. Because they decrease the rate and pumping action of the normal heart and prevent them from increasing much during exercise, beta blockers should not be used in athletes or patients who are very physically active. On the other hand, the decreased rate and work of the heart lessen its need for oxygen, which is beneficial for patients with angina (pain or pressure sensation in the chest caused by failure of oxygen to reach the heart). Therefore, **beta blockers are a good choice in patients with angina. Strong evidence also indicates that these drugs may prevent a second heart attack,** which is a compelling reason for their use following a heart attack in individuals with or without hypertension. In addition, beta blockers have proved effective in treating individuals whose hypertension appears related to an overactive sympathetic nervous system. Such individuals have rapid heart rates and considerable fluctuations of their blood pressure.

Beta blockers are almost as effective as diuretics in lowering the blood pressure of hypertensive persons. When both types of drugs are given in proper dosage, pressures can be normalized in more than 80% of patients.

Angiotensin-converting enzyme (ACE) inhibitors are newer drugs that are as effective as diuretics and beta blockers in lowering blood pressure. Except for a dry, hacking cough that appears in 10% to 20% of patients, these agents produce few side effects and rarely cause impotence. As a result, they have become very popular antihypertensive medications. **ACE inhibitors' ability to prevent or slow kidney damage in patients with diabetes, and their beneficial effects in patients with heart failure, especially if hypertension is present, or following a heart attack have further increased their popularity.** An ACE inhibitor may improve the antihypertensive effect of most antihypertensive medications, especially when it is used in combination with a diuretic.

Angiotensin II receptor blockers (A II blockers) are the newest addition to the list of antihypertensive drugs. They appear to be as effective as the ACE inhibitors but have the advantage of not causing a cough. Whether they can match all of the beneficial effects of the ACE inhibitors remains to be seen.

Calcium-channel blockers have become very popular antihypertensive drugs. Only the long-acting drugs are currently recommended, however, because short-acting calcium antagonists can cause a drop in blood pressure and increase heart rate. In addition, the short-acting drugs have been reported to increase the likelihood of heart attack in some hypertensive patients. The ability of the long-acting versions to lower blood pressure is similar to that of other antihypertensive medications. **Calcium antagonists appear particularly effective in older persons, African Americans, and sodium-sensitive individuals.** Because some of the calcium-channel blockers decrease the electrical conduction in the heart, they should be used with caution in patients who take beta blockers and in patients who already have some slowing of conduction in the heart.

Alpha$_1$ blockers are typically used when normalization of blood pressure is not achieved with a combination of the other antihypertensive drugs. These agents improve urinary flow in some men who suffer obstruction to urination due to an enlarged prostate. In addition, they also may lower total cholesterol and triglycerides and increase "good" cholesterol (HDL), and they may be useful in some physically active individuals in whom beta blockers would be contraindicated.

Alpha$_2$ agonists (which act mainly on the brain) are not usually chosen to treat hypertension because of their side effects of sedation and an annoying dry mouth. However, Aldomet is the antihypertensive drug most frequently used to treat hypertension in pregnancy, as it is effective and safe for both mother and fetus and has relatively few adverse side effects.

Combinations of alpha$_1$ and beta blockers have been available for many years and are occasionally used to treat hypertension; more recently many other combinations of antihypertensive drugs have become available (see Question 66). Furthermore, because of their convenience, combinations of two antihypertensive drugs in one pill have increased in popularity. Of course, it is impossible to determine how effective each drug is when it is given in combination, or to determine whether only one of the drugs in proper dosage might adequately normalize mild (stage 1) hypertension. Given that at least two drugs will be required to normalize blood pressure in at least 80% of patients with more severe (stage 2 or 3) hypertension and even in some mild hypertensives, starting treatment with a combination of drugs seems very reasonable. Furthermore, to lower blood pressure, small doses of each drug in combination will result in fewer side effects than a large dose of a single medication.

Rarely potent vasodilators are required in circumstances where other medications are unable to normalize the blood pressure.

Some of the older drugs (in particular, adrenergic depleters) are rarely used today because of their potential side effects and because other drugs can better control hypertension.

In summary, treatment of hypertension should be tailored to suit each patient and to ensure maximum benefits, as the drugs used in some individuals are determined by the history of a medical condition or a coexistent disease. Weight reduction for patients who are overweight or obese, limitation of salt and alcohol intake, and appropriate exercise are always indicated. Of extreme importance is cessation of cigarette smoking, as smoking can accelerate damage to the blood vessels of the heart, brain, and elsewhere (see Question 51). The presence of hypertension further increases the chance of a heart attack and stroke and of obstruction to blood flow in the legs.

Treatment of hypertension should be tailored to suit each patient and to ensure maximum benefits, as the drugs used in some individuals are determined by the history of a medical condition or a coexistent disease.

In general, treatment of an individual with mild to moderate hypertension (less than 180/120 mm Hg) and without any history or current evidence of disease can initially consist of a long-acting thiazide diuretic (water pill) or a beta blocker. If the patient has any complications of hypertension, higher blood pressures, or very severe malignant hypertension, then more aggressive treatment—sometimes requiring intravenous drugs and even hospitalization—will be needed. An ACE inhibitor or a calcium-channel blocker may also be effective as the initial treatment, although these two drug classes' ability to reduce the complications and mortality rate from hypertension has not yet been as firmly established as that of the thiazides and beta blockers. The latter two types of drugs are also available as generics, which makes them considerably less expensive than the newer drugs.

A good reason for initiating treatment with a diuretic is that perhaps 50% to 60% of hypertensives are salt-sensitive. Diuretics are especially effective in these patients, because they eliminate salt and water. They also appear to significantly enhance the effectiveness of other antihypertensive drugs—especially the ACE inhibitors. **Normalization of blood pressure to levels below 135/85 mm Hg often requires the combination of two— and occasionally three or four—drugs.**

It is impossible to predict with certainty who will respond best to a specific antihypertensive drug and who will or will not tolerate the drug, so **selection of a specific antihypertensive medication and the appropriate dosage depends somewhat on trial and observation.** Certain medical conditions may preclude the use of some antihypertensive drugs, whereas some drugs are specifically indicated with coexisting medical conditions. Consult your physician to find out when certain drugs are indicated or contraindicated (Table 10).

The ultimate goal of antihypertensive treatment is to prevent the complications of hypertension and to reduce the mortality rate by normalizing blood pressure. With the drugs available today, blood pressure can be controlled successfully in almost all patients who are motivated to work with their physician to determine the proper drug or combination of drugs and dosages for successful treatment. Specialists in hypertension should

Table 10. *Special Circumstances When Various Antihypertensive Drugs May Be Indicated or Contraindicated for Treatment of Hypertension*

Drug	Indications	Contraindications
Thiazide diuretics	• Heart failure • Salt-sensitive hypertension (especially African Americans) • Older persons (especially with only systolic hypertension) • Osteoporosis	• History of gout (painful, inflamed joint) • Impairment of kidney function
Beta blockers	• Prevention of a second heart attack • Chest pain or pressure sensation (angina) due to poor blood supply to heart • Cases where the heart muscle is excessively thick, which impairs heart function • Hyperactive heart and vascular system • Heart failure • Some irregularities of heart rhythm • Some cases with rapid heart rate due to overactive thyroid gland • Some types of hand tremor • Migraine	• Impaired electrical conduction in heart (heart block) • Very slow heart rate • Asthma and lung disease with airway obstruction (e.g., chronic bronchitis or emphysema) • Athletes and young, physically very active persons
ACE inhibitors and angiotensin II blockers	• Diabetes, especially with kidney damage • Heart failure • Following heart attack in some patients	• Pregnancy • Use with caution in patients with kidney disease, as they may retain potassium
Calcium-channel blockers	• Chest pain or pressure sensation (angina) due to poor blood supply to heart • Poor circulation in the legs • Some irregularities of heart rhythm (nondihydropyridines) • Older persons and African Americans (especially with systolic hypertension) • Migraine (nondihydropyridines)	• Use with caution in patients receiving beta blockers, as some calcium-channel blockers (nondihydropyridines) may further impair electrical conduction in the heart

Table 10. *Continued*

Drug	Indications	Contraindications
Alpha$_1$ antagonists	• Men with urination difficulty because of prostate enlargement • May decrease bad cholesterol (LDL) and triglycerides and increase good cholesterol (HDL)	• Use with caution in patients prone to fainting
Alpha$_2$ agonists	• Pregnancy, but only Aldomet is recommended • Hypertension not controlled by other drugs • Persons experiencing panic attacks and symptoms resulting from withdrawal of addictive drugs	
Direct vasodilators	• Cases where hypertension is very difficult to control (however, because they cause a rapid heart beat and water retention, a beta blocker and diuretic should be used in addition to the direct vasodilator)	
Combination alpha$_1$ and beta blocker	• Heart failure, but only Coreg (carvediol) is recommended	

be consulted regarding patients who are difficult to manage. It is a remarkable achievement that lifestyle changes and antihypertensive therapy have reduced the number of stroke and heart fatalities by 60% and 54%, respectively, in the past 25 years!

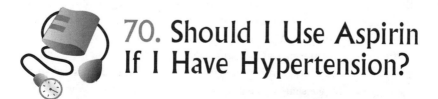

70. Should I Use Aspirin If I Have Hypertension?

Our recommendation in treating patients with hypertension is to first normalize their blood pressure. Then, if there are no contraindications (such as a history of an ulcer of the digestive tract, any bleeding tendency, sensitivity to aspirin or any of the nonsteroidal anti-inflammatory drugs (NSAIDs), or use of an anticoagulant such as coumadin), patients are started on one baby aspirin daily. This approach is especially indicated if the patient has a history of a heart attack, stroke, or transient ischemic attack (TIA—also known as a ministroke) and particularly in patients who are more than 50 years old.

In treating patients with hypertension, first normalize their blood pressure. Then, if there are no contraindications, start them on one baby aspirin daily.

Aspirin is probably the most commonly used medication in most parts of the world. Its popularity derives from its remarkable ability to combat inflammation by blocking the effect of certain hormones called prostaglandins and to reduce or eliminate all sorts of pain, whether the pain is acute and transitory or chronic, as occurs in arthritis. In addition, aspirin interferes with blood clotting by preventing platelets (very small cell-like structures in the blood) from sticking to one another, as they normally do, to help form blood clots when needed. This anticlotting effect likely explains why aspirin reduces the risk of a first heart attack, improves survival of patients who have had a heart attack, and reduces the chance of another heart attack by as much as 50%. Furthermore, this drug reduces the chance of heart attack and death in patients with chest pain or pressure sensation (angina) due to poor circulation to the heart muscle.

One recent study demonstrated that one regular aspirin [325 milligrams (mg)] taken every other day by healthy men can decrease the number of heart attacks. The same study also indicated that aspirin may not reduce the occurrence of stroke and brain damage occurring for the first time. Furthermore, it may increase the mortality rate in patients with hemorrhagic stroke. On the other hand, evidence indicates that aspirin can reduce by 20% the occurrence of stroke in individuals who have already had a nonhemorrhagic stroke or a TIA that resulted from a clot formation in a vessel supplying blood to the brain. Some strokes result from hemorrhage in the brain—aspirin should not be used if there is any evidence of such bleeding, as it might increase the bleeding.

Blood clots may form in vessels of the brain that become narrowed by atherosclerosis (hardening of the arteries due to excessive accumulation of cholesterol), or clots formed elsewhere in the body (such as in the large arteries of the neck or in the heart) may travel in the circulation and reach the brain, where they can block the circulation and cause brain damage. Aspirin may reduce the chance that such clots will form; however, to prevent clots in the heart produced by an irregular heart beat (atrial fibrillation), another anticlotting agent (coumadin) is used that is more effective than aspirin.

Aspirin may irritate the lining of the stomach and intestinal tract and cause some bleeding. It may also aggravate or cause ulceration, sometimes with severe bleeding. Therefore, patients with ulcers or those who develop abdominal complaints such as pain or "indigestion" should not use aspirin or similar anti-inflammatory drugs—for example, Advil, Motrin, Nuprin, Naprosyn, Indocin, Clinoril, Ansaid, Aleve, or other so-called nonsteroidal anti-inflammatory drugs (NSAIDs). Smaller doses of aspirin, such as a baby aspirin (81 mg/day), may be just as effective or more effective than a regular aspirin (325 mg/day) in preventing heart attacks and strokes due to blood clots. A possible explanation for

Patients with ulcers or those who develop abdominal complaints such as pain or "indigestion" should not use aspirin or similar anti-inflammatory drugs.

this phenomenon is that lower doses of aspirin can block the aggregation (sticking together) of platelets by thromboxane, a hormone that makes platelets more sticky and causes blood vessels to constrict. Both effects are undesirable, because they would promote the formation of a clot. On the other hand, a low dose of aspirin does not inhibit formation of prostacycline, a hormone that prevents platelet stickiness, promotes dilation of blood vessels, and thereby prevents clot formation.

NSAIDs, when taken repeatedly and especially for prolonged periods, may reduce the effectiveness of diuretics (water pills) because their effect on the kidney can cause salt and water retention. Furthermore, they can decrease the production of hormones that dilate blood vessels and reduce the effectiveness of various drugs used to lower blood pressure. When taken only occasionally, NSAIDs do not interfere with blood pressure control. **Aspirin does not seem to interfere significantly with blood pressure control of hypertensive patients, unlike most other NSAIDs, when used repeatedly in large amounts.**

A final possible benefit associated with taking aspirin regularly is that several reputable studies have reported that this practice may reduce the frequency of colon cancer by 50%!

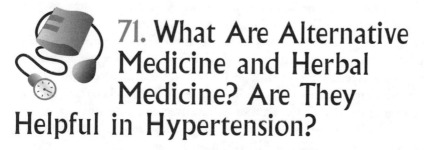

71. What Are Alternative Medicine and Herbal Medicine? Are They Helpful in Hypertension?

It is unfortunate that a large percentage of the public is so easily influenced by unsubstantiated health claims of the benefits of alternative treatment of their medical problems. The excessive barrage of these claims through newspapers, magazines, TV, radio, health-food stores, and the Internet, and the vigorous endorsement of alternative medical approaches on talk shows and by friends and acquaintances can often overwhelm and convince an extraordinary number of Americans to use these alternatives.

In his book *Good News About High Blood Pressure*, Dr. Tom Pickering has addressed the flaws and dangers of accepting alternative forms of medical therapy. By definition, "alternative medicine" (also known as "complementary" or "extended" medicine) involves the use of unproved therapeutic procedures, which are not generally advocated or employed by the vast majority of the medical profession. These procedures include chelation therapy, homeopathy, acupuncture, chiropractic treatment, massage, biofeedback, meditation, herbs, and nutritional supplements. In 1997, an estimated 42% of Americans participated in unconventional (alternative) treatment at a cost of $27 billion, most of which took the form of out-of-pocket expenses! Hypertension was among the top 10 conditions for which individuals used alternative therapy, without consulting their physician. There is no convincing evidence that alternative medicine can control hypertension.

There is no convincing evidence that alternative medicine can control hypertension.

Any claim that some form of alternative medicine can cure a large variety of medical conditions is reminiscent of the tales spun by old-time "medicine men" who traveled about the country, promising miraculous cures for almost any ailment by consuming a mysterious tonic. Obviously, no single cure exists for so many different ailments! Unfortunately, some may push forms of alternative medicine that are unproved and even hazardous to the patient. For instance, claims have been made that chelation therapy, homeopathy, and chiropractic treatments can lower blood pressure, even though there is no scientific proof of these claims.

Chelation makes use of a chemical named EDTA (ethylenediaminetetraacetic acid), which is given intravenously to cleanse the blood. This technique can be an effective form of treatment for lead poisoning. As pointed out by Dr. Pickering, however, claims that it can reduce hardening of the arteries and blood pressure; normalize weight; lessen arthritis; reverse impotence, hair loss, and Alzheimer's disease; prevent chronic fatigue; reduce cancer mortality by 90%; and produce a youthful appearance are simply ridiculous. Pickering further notes that chelation can lower calcium in the blood and result in serious irregularities of the heart, cause respiratory arrest, muscle spasms, and kidney damage. Indeed, some patients have died as a result of chelation therapy.

Homeopathy is a therapeutic approach to treating disease that was originally developed by Dr. Samuel Hahnemann (1755–1843). He proposed that certain drugs, which in ordinary amounts produce symptoms and signs or manifestations of a disease in healthy subjects, should be used in very small amounts to treat patients with that disease. Although some physicians endorse this approach, it seems very unlikely that the extremely small doses of drugs used in homeopathy would have any significant effect on a disease process. It is well recognized that the effectiveness of most drugs depends on adequate dosage. Thus it is unreasonable to believe that the tiny doses employed in homeopathy can cause some therapeutic, physiologic, pharmacologic, or biochemical event that can alter a disease process. Little evidence has been published to validate or scientifically support homeopathic therapy for any disease, including hypertension.

Approximately 12 million acupuncture treatments are performed each year in the United States. Acupuncture appears to have some beneficial therapeutic applications, particularly in the realm of treatment of pain and addiction. Some reports describe patients who have undergone abdominal surgical procedures with acupuncture but no anesthesia and who did not experience any severe pain during surgical incisions. The success of acupuncture in the treatment of pain remains poorly understood; practitioners claim that inserting thin needles in certain areas of the body may stimulate nerves that send impulses to the spinal cord and brain and suppress pain pathways. Because pain severity is a subjective, difficult-to-measure sensation, there is no easy or scientific way to evaluate acupuncture's effectiveness. In some cases, improvement may reflect a placebo effect. Although some claim that acupuncture can lower high blood pressure and raise low blood pressure, no good evidence supports these claims.

Chiropractic treatments concentrate mainly on manipulations of the spine in an attempt to correct misalignment of vertebrae, thereby relieving pressure on nerves and restoring normal nerve conduction to muscles and various organs of the body. Again, claims about chiropractic treatment are difficult to verify. Relief of some types of pain may occur due to a placebo effect in some cases. Claims that chiropractic treatment is beneficial for a variety of diseases (unrelated to the spine or muscles) and that it can lower blood pressure are unfounded.

Another very popular form of alternative medicine is the "natural" cure, which involves a large variety of healthy food supplements and herbal remedies. Some very important drugs were initially discovered in natural sources—for example, aspirin was found in willow tree bark; digitalis was present in the foxglove plant; a blood thinner was found in clover; and Reserpine, a blood-pressure-lowering drug, was isolated from an Indian root. Garlic, when consumed in large amounts, may lower "bad" cholesterol and raise "good" cholesterol (see Questions 50, 73); although a few reports claim that it may lower blood pressure when taken in large amounts, most studies indicate that it has no such effect. Virtually none of the commonly used herbs, which can be obtained in food stores, have been scientifically evaluated to determine their action, potency, and safety.

Though very widely available, herbal remedies can cause many harmful side effects, including death and serious interaction with prescription drugs (see Question 73). One should be aware of the hazards of these supplements and herbal remedies, and consult a physician before using them (see Table 11 on page 125).

Finally, we should mention copper bracelets and magnets, which are purported to relieve all sorts of pain. Many persons will swear this simple alternative medicine brings enormous benefits or cure of a chronic pain. Magnets are usually placed in the bed under the mattress and, following one night's sleep, miraculous cures of backaches have been reported. Unfortunately, no scientific studies have documented these anecdotal reports—that is, no studies have compared the beneficial effects of magnets with similar-appearing objects that have no magnetic properties. Such a study is essential to evaluate the validity of these items. This form of alternative medicine has no place in the treatment of hypertension, and it is important that patients with heart pacemakers avoid close contact with strong magnets!

In conclusion, if you are considering alternative medicine, we strongly urge you to consult your physician before using any such therapeutic remedy, as some may be very harmful or even lethal. **To repeat our earlier statement, there is no good evidence that alternative medicine has significant value in the treatment of hypertension.** For instance, reports that garlic, in large amounts, can lower blood pressure in some hypertensive individuals have recently been refuted.

In reality, the benefits of alternative medicine may depend mainly on the "placebo effect." A placebo (derived from Latin, meaning "I will please") is defined as a "dummy medical treatment": a medicinal preparation or treatment that has no specific pharmacologic activity against the patient's illness or complaint (see Question 74). A beneficial effect from a dummy treatment is best explained by the psychophysiological effects experienced by the patient who has high expectation for improvement. Today nearly 64% of medical schools offer courses in alternative medicine, and it is important that physicians and patients familiarize themselves with the flaws and especially the dangers of alternative medicine.

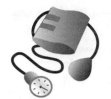

72. Are Relaxation and Biofeedback Techniques Effective in Hypertension Management?

Some members of the public continue to believe that relaxation and biofeedback techniques can be of therapeutic value in the management of essential hypertension, the commonest form of hypertension for which the cause remains unknown. In reality, these techniques do not improve hypertension.

A number of relaxation procedures may improve a person's sense of well-being and relieve tension and nervousness. In essence, these techniques are a form of stress management, and they depend, to a major extent, on the relaxation of major muscles of the body. In addition, hypnosis (a state of a deep relaxation and altered consciousness), Zen meditation, yoga, and transcendental meditation require mental concentration ("to clear the mind of all distractions") and sometimes the repetition of a word or sound by the individual. Relaxation may be so pronounced that brain wave studies (electroencephalogram changes) indicate a pattern similar to that seen during sleep. As a result of this profound degree of relaxation, the activity of the nervous system diminishes. The decrease in sympathetic nerve activity is accompanied by a slowing of the heart rate and a dilation of arteries, which results in a modest degree of blood pressure reduction. Unfortunately, this reduction is only transitory and is not maintained for long.

Biofeedback is designed to help an individual sense or feel a change in a bodily function, such as heart rate and blood pressure. Using instrumentation that can convey information about blood pressure, heart rate, or the degree of muscle contraction to the individual participating in biofeedback, the late Dr. Alvin Shapiro (an authority on hypertension and stress) reported that systolic and diastolic pressures may be reduced by as much as 20 and 10 mm Hg, respectively.

It is very apparent that stress results in elevation of blood pressure, whereas mental and muscular relaxation are accompanied by a decrease in blood pressure. For example, Dr. Tom Pickering, using an instrument that monitors blood pressure for 24 hours, found that most individuals' blood pressure is about 5 mm Hg higher while at work than it is when they are more relaxed at home in the evening.

Unfortunately, the lowering of blood pressure achievable with relaxation techniques and biofeedback is only temporary. After terminating one or a series of these procedures, blood pressure returns promptly to the level present before the relaxation or biofeedback procedures began. It must be concluded that these techniques, although of interest experimentally, have no therapeutic value in the long-term management of hypertension.

73. Are Health-Food Supplements, Herbal Remedies, and "Body Builders" Good for You? Can They Affect Your Blood Pressure, and Can They Be Harmful?

A frenetic and irrational craze for health-food supplements and herbal remedies has developed throughout the United States in the past few decades. In 1998, 60 million Americans spent nearly $4 billion on these products, and demand for them continues to increase dramatically. **No regulation of the quality and strength of herbal remedies has been established. Although some have been helpful, others may be harmful and cause serious interactions with some prescription drugs.** In 1999, the Food and Drug Administration began requiring manufacturers to include labels indicating the part of the plant used in herbal remedies.

Table 11 lists some popular health-food supplements and herbal remedies and their side effects, as reported by the Mayo Clinic. For instance, a variety of "natural" diuretics have been advocated to increase the elimination of salt and water, even though no evidence shows that they are efficacious in lowering blood pressure. In addition, soy protein in large amounts may decrease "bad" cholesterol but has no effect on blood pressure.

In the October 12, 1999, *New York Times*, a lengthy article—"Side Effects Raise Flag on Dangers of Ephedra"—discussed the merits of one popular herbal remedy. Ephedra, which is also known as ma huang, is derived from a shrub-like plant that is prevalent in Asia. Some claim that it curbs appetite, elevates metabolism, burns fat, increases energy, improves muscle tone, sharpens sex performance, and improves concentration. Glowing accounts on the Internet have unfortunately raised expectations that ephedra will be a remarkable solution for many physical problems.

Table 11. *Selected Food Supplements and Their Purported Health Claims*

Food Supplements Promoted as Lowering Blood Pressure	Comment
Coenzyme Q-10	No good evidence it lowers blood pressure.
Gingko biloba	No good evidence it lowers blood pressure.
Green tea	No good evidence it lowers blood pressure.
Vitamin C	No good evidence it lowers blood pressure.
Omega-3 polyunsaturated fatty acids (fish oil)	Large doses may lower blood pressure (and triglycerides, but have little if any effect on cholesterol) and can reduce blood clotting.
Garlic	Large doses can lower "bad" cholesterol without changing good cholesterol. Garlic does not lower blood pressure.

Supplements Promoted as Increasing Blood Pressure	Comment
Ephedrine (ephedra)	Can cause a dangerous rise in blood pressure.
Licorice root	Can increase blood pressure.
Yohimbine	Can increase blood pressure.

Herbal Remedy	Potential Side Effects
Aloe	Increased toxicity of some drugs used to treat heart failure and cause abdominal cramps.
Echinacea	Suppression of the immune system.
Feverfew	Interaction with anticoagulants to increase bleeding.
Gingko biloba	Bleeding in eye if given with aspirin, bleeding in the brain; inhibition of blood clotting.
Ginseng	Nervousness, excitement, headache, insomnia, and palpitations. May elevate blood pressure. May cause falsely elevated digoxin blood levels and mislead physician with inappropriate treatment.
Kava-kava	Muscle weakness; skin discoloration.
Saw palmetto	Diarrhea; upset stomach.
St. John's wort	May augment depression, if the user is taking an antidepressant; sun sensitivity; interactions with blood pressure drugs. Can decrease the effectiveness of medications for AIDS and heart transplants.
Valeriana	Sedative effect causing drowsiness.
Ma huang	Stroke, heart attack, rapid heart rate, and sudden death.
Comfrey	Liver failure.
Aristolochia fangchi	Kidney failure; cancer of the urinary tract.

The fact that ephedra's main ingredient is ephedrine makes this herbal "remedy" a potentially very dangerous substance. Like amphetamine, it can stimulate the nervous system and produce side effects including hypertension, a rapid heart rate, anxiety, insomnia, psychosis, heart attack, stroke, and death. Obviously, the public is not fully aware of the serious risks of consuming excess amounts of ephedra, as this year's sales of one ephedra-containing product may reach $900 million. According to the *New York Times* article, use of "ephedrine-based products is 'rampant among athletes,' even though it has been banned by the National Collegiate Athletic Association and the U.S. Olympic Committee."

Ephedra's main ingredient—ephedrine— renders this herbal "remedy" a potentially very dangerous substance. Like amphetamine, it can stimulate the nervous system and produce side effects including hypertension, a rapid heart rate, anxiety, insomnia, psychosis, heart attack, stroke, and death.

Although many over-the-counter drugs contain ephedrine, the concentration of ephedrine is indicated on the packaging and the drugs are regulated by the Food and Drug Administration. Thus guidance on the use of these drugs is always available. In contrast, the concentration of ephedrine in ephedra preparations may vary considerably and be dangerous to consume, especially in large amounts.

The use of "body builders" such as anabolic steroids or GHB (gammahydroxybutyrate) may cause severe illness, and occasionally death. Steroids have not been shown to improve athletic performance, but may cause retention of salt and water, which can elevate blood pressure. Furthermore, they may markedly decrease HDL (high-density lipoprotein, the "good" cholesterol).

No one should risk using herbal products about which they know little or nothing. Herbal products are often spiked with drugs not listed on the labels and sometimes contain lead, arsenic, or mercury contaminants. *Please* check with your physician before using herbal remedies and health food supplements. Do not use body builders at all. Do not experiment with your health!

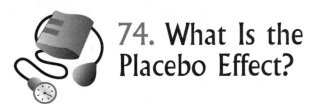

74. What Is the Placebo Effect?

A placebo is defined as an inert, inactive, innocuous, harmless substance, or a dummy medical treatment, which has no effect on bodily functions. It is used as a control when evaluating the therapeutic effectiveness of a drug or procedure (see Questions 7, 71). The word "placebo" actually means "I shall please." Often an inert substance with no pharmacologically active ingredients (such as a sugar or starch pill), when ingested, can appear to exert various beneficial effects—a phenomenon known as the placebo effect. Therefore, to establish the benefit of a drug or procedure, the therapeutic efficacy of the proposed treatment must be significantly greater than that of a placebo.

Often an inert substance with no pharmacologically active ingredients, when ingested, can appear to exert various beneficial effects—a phenomenon known as the placebo effect.

It is important that neither the patient nor the physician administering a drug or placebo knows which is the drug and which is the placebo. Such a double-blind study eliminates any bias by the patient or physician in analyzing and assessing results of a drug evaluation.

Perhaps not surprisingly, placebos have been shown to reduce systolic blood pressure by 5 to 10 mm Hg and diastolic blood pressure by 3 to 5 mm Hg; they can also cause "side effects" such as headache, sexual dysfunction, weakness, fatigue, and dizziness. In some comparative trials, the placebo caused just as many side effects as the active drug and, in some instances, even more side effects!

Expectations about and anticipation of a benefit from any substance or procedure can result in a significant placebo effect, regardless of whether the drug or procedure has any real therapeutic value. The warmth and caring shown by a sympathetic physician can create a patient–physician relationship that raises the patient's hopes and improves his or her mood and well-being. As a result, a good patient–physician relationship can contribute to the placebo effect. Obviously, the psychological effects from the combination of a placebo and a warm and close relationship with a caring physician may be considerable, sometimes causing the patient to feel much improved.

Even an abnormal objective finding, such as an elevated blood pressure, may improve with the use of some innocuous but awesome-looking machine that impresses the patient by harmlessly emitting sounds and lights, which the patient believes are therapeutic. Repeated treatments with such a dramatically impressive device were reported by the late Dr. William Goldring, an authority on hypertension, and his colleagues at New York University Medical Center to cause a pronounced lowering of blood pressure by the placebo effect. Hypertension invariably returned to pretreatment levels after this treatment was discontinued, however. This placebo effect most likely resulted from reduced emotional tension and probably a decreased activity of the sympathetic nervous system, which resulted in dilation of arteries and reduction of the blood pressure. According to Dr. Herbert Spiegel, the placebo effect can occur "when conditions are optimal for hope, faith, trust, and love."

The power of suggestion from friends and acquaintances that a certain procedure or herbal remedy may relieve a variety of symptoms or conditions may have dramatic effects. Infinite anecdotal claims and testimonials have been made about alternative forms of treatment (see Question 71), suggesting that such remedies can result in miraculous cures of even long-standing medical problems. For example, claims have been made that chronic backaches may sometimes be cured by sleeping on a bed with magnets placed beneath the mattress. Those claiming cures of their backaches are absolutely convinced that the magnets were responsible for the cure. Although this explanation seems highly unlikely, we can test this theory by placing magnets under the mattresses of one series of beds and nonmagnetized objects, which appear identical to the magnets, under the mattresses of another series of beds. Individuals with backaches can then report any benefit from sleeping in these beds. If essentially no significant difference is seen in backache improvement between those sleeping over magnets versus those sleeping in beds with nonmagnetized objects, then any improvement must be attributed to a placebo effect.

The importance of understanding and recognizing the placebo effect cannot be overstated. In the final analysis, one must appreciate the significance of the placebo effect before accepting any unproved form of treatment as being responsible for a therapeutic effect. The public should be alerted to recognize that benefits from various types of alternative medicine, herbal remedies, and "health" foods (see Questions 71, 73) may result from a placebo effect, rather than from any medicinal action. One must also remember that the use of some alternative medicines, herbs, and health foods can actually be harmful.

75. Are Vitamins Helpful in Treating People with Hypertension and Hypercholesterolemia? Can They Be Harmful?

The interest of the public in vitamins has increased enormously in recent years, reflecting the strong belief that some vitamins are valuable in treating a variety of diseases. Although the claims of health benefits may be overzealous, very compelling evidence does show that people who consume large amounts of fruits and vegetables have less cancer and heart disease. Some also claim, but have not yet proved, that vitamin C (ascorbic acid) and vitamin E (alpha-tocopherol)—both of which are antioxidants—may prevent arterial damage and the deleterious effects from harmful oxidation products known as super-oxides (see Question 96). Therefore, it seems reasonable to eat more fruits and vegetables and to take a multivitamin tablet on a daily basis. In addition, 400 international units (IU) of vitamin E is recommended as a possible protection against hardening of the arteries (atherosclerosis), as only large doses of this vitamin have proved effective as an antioxidant; dietary intake plus a multivitamin provide far less than the recommended antioxidant dose of vitamin E. The possible protection from atherosclerosis provided by vitamin C and E may be helpful in reducing the arterial damage caused by hypertension and hypercholesterolemia.

> *Vitamin C (ascorbic acid) and vitamin E (alpha-tocopherol)—both antioxidants—are claimed to prevent arterial damage and the deleterious effects from harmful oxidation products known as superoxides. Vitamin E has no effect on blood pressure or blood lipids, whereas vitamin C may lower blood cholesterol and pressure to a minor extent.*

Vitamin E has no effect on blood pressure or blood lipids (cholesterol and triglycerides), even when consumed in large amounts. Megadoses are not toxic, but there is no need to use more than 400 IU daily to obtain its possible beneficial antioxidant effect.

Vitamin C may lower blood cholesterol and pressure, but these changes are relatively minor, and daily supplements of 500 milligrams (mg) appear necessary to achieve these effects. There is no reason to take large amounts of vitamin C to lower cholesterol or blood pressure, as this substance is only minimally effective in reducing cholesterol and does not lower blood pressure. One recent report indicated that persons who consume at least 480 mg of vitamin C daily developed arterial thickening, which was almost three times greater than the arterial thickening seen in individuals not taking vitamin C. Additional studies are needed to confirm this finding.

Although there has been much talk about the ability of large doses (megadoses) of vitamin C to prevent the common cold, this claim has been scientifically investigated and never substantiated. Furthermore, megadoses of more than 1000 mg can cause kidney stones, increase blood levels of estrogen in women taking estrogen, interfere with absorption of vitamin B_{12}, and cause scurvy in the offspring of some mothers on megadoses.

Niacin (vitamin B_3, nicotinic acid) can effectively lower "bad" cholesterol (LDL—low-density lipoprotein), elevate "good" cholesterol (HDL—high-density lipoprotein), and reduce triglycerides. All of these lipid (fat) changes can help prevent or minimize atherosclerosis (damaging of the lining of arteries), thereby reducing and possibly reversing impairment of blood flow to vital organs. As with other drugs that lower LDL cholesterol, mortality from heart attacks may be reduced. **Niacin does not, however, lower blood pressure.** Unfortunately, its use to treat lipid abnormalities is frequently accompanied by a number of side effects, such as flushing, itching, intestinal upsets, stomach ulcers, gout (due to increased uric acid), difficulty of blood sugar control in diabetics (because niacin increases blood sugar), aggravation of asthma, and impairment of liver function, sometimes with jaundice. Rarely a pronounced transitory decrease in blood pressure may occur. The combination of aspirin with niacin can reduce flushing and itching, which are the two most common and annoying side effects. Niacin probably should not be used in patients with heart disease or diabetes. Because so many other drugs are available that can effectively treat abnormalities of blood fats with few side effects, we prefer to initially use other medications for this indication.

Folic acid is valuable in preventing atherosclerosis, apparently working by preventing elevated blood levels of homocysteine (an amino acid—a substance that builds protein). Given that an estimated 40% of the U.S. population consumes deficient amounts of folic acid, it would seem prudent for Americans to consume more folic acid in the form of one-a-day vitamins. **Folic acid does not have any effect on blood pressure, cholesterol, or triglycerides.**

Other vitamins do not appear to have any effect in treating hypertension or hypercholesterolemia. It is noteworthy, however, that toxic doses of vitamin D may significantly increase calcium in the blood, which might then cause hypertension.

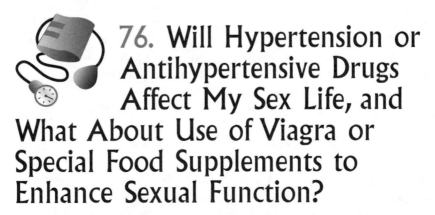

76. Will Hypertension or Antihypertensive Drugs Affect My Sex Life, and What About Use of Viagra or Special Food Supplements to Enhance Sexual Function?

Hypertension alone (without any complications) may affect your sex life, with impaired sexual function sometimes improving after blood pressure is reduced with antihypertensive drugs. Nevertheless, impotence or a lack of desire for sex (libido) is often psychogenic in origin (that is, due to mental and emotional attitude). Low blood pressure may also be a cause of impotence, especially in older men who have impaired blood supply to the penis due to atherosclerosis of the arteries. Failure to adequately perform sexual intercourse can cause considerable anxiety and depression in men and can cause disappointment and even anger in the spouse, which can lead to a disturbed relationship.

Sexual dysfunction (inability to obtain and maintain an erection) has been reported to affect 50% of normotensive men between the ages of 40 to 70. It is conceivable that this rate of dysfunction might be even greater in hypertensive males on no medications, as concern over the presence of hypertension could cause additional anxiety and further compound the problem. As noted above, impotence is often caused by psychogenic problems, although atherosclerosis with impairment of blood flow to the penis is also a common cause. In addition, conditions that damage the nerves (such as diabetes) that control the erectile function of the penis, as well as a deficiency of the male hormone testosterone, may lead to sexual dysfunction. Abnormal blood flow problems in the penis can be accurately identified by Doppler ultrasonography and deficiency of testosterone can be determined by a blood test.

Most antihypertensive drugs probably do not cause impotence. Diuretics and beta blockers may rarely be responsible for sexual dysfunction in men, but no remarkable change in sexual performance was experienced in men or women taking alpha₁ blockers, ACE inhibitors, or calcium-channel blockers. The exception was Norvasc, which caused sexual dysfunction in about 2% of patients. (Some of the older sympathetic-nerve-blocking drugs may interfere with sexual function, but they are very rarely used to treat hypertension today. Aldactone is very rarely used to treat essential hypertension, but recently was found to help some patients with congestive heart failure; it can cause enlargement of the breasts in men and loss of sex desire.) In the event that the patient believes an antihypertensive drug has decreased sexual function, the drug may be discontinued by the physician, if necessary, and another drug used. In most cases, however, the antihypertensive medication will probably not be the root cause of the impotence.

Most antihypertensive drugs probably do not cause impotence. Diuretics and beta blockers may rarely be responsible for sexual dysfunction in men, but no remarkable change in sexual performance was experienced in men or women taking alpha₁ blockers, ACE inhibitors, or calcium-channel blockers.

Sexual dysfunction has not been as well studied in women as it has been in men. Some women experienced a decrease in libido and/or lack of orgasmic response during intercourse after taking some of the drugs that were used to lower blood pressure in the past. None of the currently used medications to treat hypertension appear to cause sexual dysfunction in women, however.

Viagra, which dilates blood vessels and improves blood flow to the penis by enhancing the effect of nitric oxide, can be used in patients with hypertension that is adequately controlled with medication or lifestyle changes. Its use may be contraindicated in patients with coronary heart disease, especially in those who have angina, a history of recent heart attack, or congestive heart failure. **Furthermore, Viagra should never be prescribed to patients taking nitrates (those used to dilate arteries, e.g., nitroglycerine, Nitro-Bid, Nitrostat, Nitrol, Nitro-Dur, Isordil, Sorbitate, Dilatrate, Imdur, Ismo, Cardilate, and others), as this combination may cause a dangerous decrease in blood pressure.** If this drug proves ineffective in restoring sexual function, then a physician specializing in this type of disorder should be consulted.

No scientific evidence has shown that any food supplements are helpful in restoring sexual function.

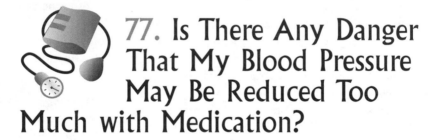

77. Is There Any Danger That My Blood Pressure May Be Reduced Too Much with Medication?

It is highly unlikely that antihypertensive medications will lead to too-low blood pressure. Indeed, it is much more likely that your blood pressure will not be reduced enough to protect you fully from the bad consequences of high blood pressure. A recent survey indicated that only 27% of the 50 million hypertensives in the United States had their blood pressure controlled to 140/90 mm Hg or less.

Some older medications, most of which are not prescribed today, had a greater effect on blood pressure in the standing position than pressure in the sitting or reclining position. They might therefore produce light-headedness or even fainting when patients stood up rapidly. **Most currently prescribed medications do not reduce blood pressure excessively in the standing position.** Rarely, when an alpha$_1$-blocking drug is first used, the patient may experience a pronounced fall of the blood pressure on standing. This problem can be avoided by taking the medication at bedtime, when the patient is recumbent and can get up cautiously if necessary. Fortunately, a drop in blood pressure on standing occurs only occasionally with the first dose and not with subsequent doses. Sometimes the physician will measure blood pressure in both the standing and sitting or reclining positions, before and after the patient has started medication, to see whether any excessive lowering of the blood pressure occurs on standing.

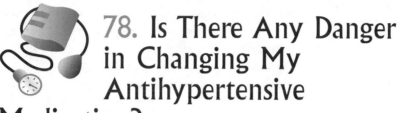

78. Is There Any Danger in Changing My Antihypertensive Medication?

Changing your antihypertensive medication should not create problems if the change is made under the supervision of your physician. Many times, if your blood pressure is not well controlled, adding or substituting blood pressure medications will bring the blood pressure down. **You should never stop a medication entirely without consulting your doctor** (see Question 66). Abrupt cessation of a beta blocker in a patient with coronary artery disease, for example, may sometimes aggravate chest pain or pressure sensation (angina) or even cause a heart attack. Suddenly discontinuing a relatively high dose of Catapress may occasionally cause a significant elevation of blood pressure.

If undesirable side effects are the reason for changing medication, be sure to discuss the problem with your doctor. Sometimes using multiple medications in small doses will reduce or eliminate side effects and control the blood pressure more effectively than using single agents.

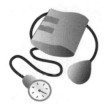

79. Why Is Hypertension Sometimes Resistant to Treatment?

Hypertension is not considered "resistant" to treatment until you have taken at least three drugs, all from different classes, including a diuretic (see Table 9 on page 102). Generally, when high blood pressure does not respond to a good combination of drugs, patients are not taking the medications as prescribed. Eating too much salt, drinking too much alcohol or taking large amounts of a nonsteroidal anti-inflammatory drug (NSAID) such as ibuprofen may also make high blood pressure less responsive to treatment. Obese patients are more likely to be resistant to treatment than are thin patients, although the culprit may actually be falsely high readings taken in the obese arm.

Hypertension is not considered "resistant" to treatment until you have taken at least three drugs, all from different classes, including a diuretic.

When blood pressure remains high despite a good combination of drugs, one should suspect that some secondary form of hypertension is present. In these cases, the problem may follow from disease in a kidney artery, blocking the flow of blood to the kidney, a tumor of the adrenal gland (pheochromocytoma or aldosteronoma), or advanced kidney disease with kidney failure (see Question 38).

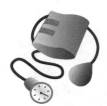

80. Can Hypertension Cause Pain in My Legs When I Walk?

Hypertension can cause leg pain if it is associated with significant damage to the arteries supplying blood to the legs. Pain, ache, or fatigue that occurs in the legs, especially in the calf muscles, on walking and then subsides with rest is usually caused by impaired blood supply to the lower extremities. This type of pain, which is called intermittent claudication, results from atherosclerotic changes (that is, hardening of the arteries with obstruction to blood flow). Impairment of blood flow may also sometimes occur above the legs and cause pain in the hip, buttock, and thigh muscles on walking. If obstruction to blood flow is very severe, then the patient may experience pain in the affected legs or feet, even when at rest. Surgical procedures may be able to improve blood supply to the legs, but occasionally amputation of a foot or leg may be necessary with severely impaired blood supply and the development of gangrene. This latter complication occurs most commonly in diabetic patients.

In addition to hypertension, risk factors for the development of atherosclerosis include cigarette smoking, high levels of "bad" cholesterol (LDL—low-density lipoprotein) and low levels of "good" cholesterol (HDL—high-density lipoprotein), and diabetes mellitus. All of these risk factors can markedly enhance the occurrence of intermittent claudication, coronary disease (atherosclerosis of the coronary arteries in the heart), cerebrovascular disease (atherosclerosis of the arteries of the brain), and atherosclerotic changes in other important arteries, such as the carotid arteries of the neck (which supply blood to the brain) and the aorta (the largest artery, which carries blood away from the heart to all parts of the body). In general, the severity of the risk factors and their number are strongly correlated with the degree of atherosclerosis and its complications. Furthermore, because all these complications occur with aging, it is extremely important to control modifiable risk factors as soon as they are recognized. Cessation of smoking is imperative (see Questions 51, 52). In addition, every effort should be made to normalize an elevated blood pressure and LDL with lifestyle changes and medication, if necessary, and to control diabetes.

Leg pains (cramps) during exercise may result from a decreased level of potassium in the body. This condition can be easily identified by measuring the concentration of potassium in the blood. Leg cramps may also occur without exercise, especially at night. The cause of these leg cramps is not clear, and there is no consistently effective treatment for them. None of those cramps are related to essential hypertension.

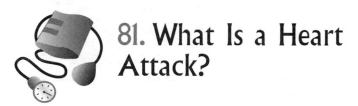

81. What Is a Heart Attack?

The term "heart attack" typically means a myocardial infarction, although it is sometimes used to describe impending infarction or spells of rapid or irregular heart beats. "Infarction" means death of some of the heart muscle, usually due to blockage of a coronary artery supplying that area of muscle. Myocardial infarction can often be prevented by appropriate treatment of hypertension. Even in patients who have already experienced a heart attack, it is possible to prolong life and prevent recurrent heart attacks by appropriately treating high blood pressure, usually with a beta blocker, an ACE inhibitor, or both.

A heart attack is, of course, an acute emergency that your physician will want to treat as soon as possible. You should immediately report to your physician any pain or sensation of pressure or tightness in the chest that persists for more than 20 to 30 minutes. Sometimes the pain is very severe and may extend into the back and neck or down the arms; it may be accompanied by sweating, nausea, and sometimes vomiting. If you cannot reach your physician, take one regular aspirin (unless you are allergic to aspirin) and go to the nearest emergency room.

Angina (chest pain, pressure sensation, or tightness, sometimes with extension of pain down the left arm) is also caused by impaired blood supply to the heart. There is no death of heart muscle, however, and the symptoms are generally less severe and usually last for fewer than 20 minutes.

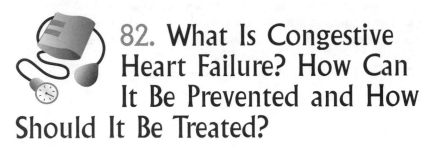

82. What Is Congestive Heart Failure? How Can It Be Prevented and How Should It Be Treated?

Heart failure occurs when the heart cannot pump blood effectively to the tissues of the body. When the pumping action becomes significantly impaired, blood backs up in the lungs, causing congestive heart failure. A number of conditions may cause congestive heart failure:

- Hypertension
- Damage to heart valves caused by infection
- Destruction of heart muscle caused by impaired blood supply, often as the result of a heart attack due to atherosclerosis and a blood clot in one of the coronary (heart) arteries
- Destruction of heart muscle due to infections, excess alcohol consumption, and other causes
- Congenital (inherited) abnormalities of the heart, its valves, or its blood vessels

Heart failure occurs when the heart cannot pump blood effectively to the tissues of the body. When the pumping action becomes significantly impaired, blood backs up in the lungs, causing congestive heart failure.

Hypertension is present in an estimated 91% of patients who develop congestive heart failure. Indeed, hypertension is the major preventable factor in this very serious condition that claims 400,000 lives annually. Frequently the muscle fibers of the left ventricle (the muscular pumping chamber of the heart) become enlarged in response to the increased work required to maintain an adequate blood flow against an elevated blood pressure; this enlargement of the heart muscle is known as left ventricular hypertrophy (LVH) (see Question 83). Similarly, hypertrophy of skeletal muscles in the biceps of the arms or elsewhere occurs with repeated demand for increased muscular work, such as weightlifting exercise. With continuation and usually worsening of untreated hypertension, the heart muscle becomes incapable of carrying out the excess work required to effectively pump blood to the tissues. At this point, congestive heart failure develops.

Adequate treatment of hypertension can markedly reduce mortality from stroke, heart attack, and congestive heart failure. Sadly, only 27% of the hypertensive population have their blood pressure under proper control. This poor success rate mainly reflects the fact that many hypertensives are unaware that they have hypertension or are receiving inadequate antihypertensive medication. The incidence of congestive heart failure is increasing in the United States partly because of aging of the population, as older people are more apt to have hypertension and atherosclerosis. This disease is the fourth most common cause for hospitalization of adults and the most common hospital discharge diagnosis for Medicare patients (patients 65 years or older).

Every effort should be made to detect hypertension as early as possible so that it can be managed appropriately. In addition, smoking cessation, weight and cholesterol control, and adequate exercise can help prevent the development of atherosclerosis and heart disease. **Congestive heart failure is an ominous manifestation, which requires hospitalization and usually treatment with ACE inhibitors or angiotensin II receptor blockers (drugs that help prevent the deleterious effects of angiotensin), diuretics (including Aldactone), salt limitation, digitalis, and sometimes other drugs to control serious heart irregularities.** Mitigation of risk factors—smoking, diabetes, hypertension, excess weight, elevated LDL (low-density lipoprotein, i.e., "bad" cholesterol) and triglycerides, sedentary lifestyle, and excess sodium in the diet—are key to preventing or reducing the occurrence of congestive heart failure.

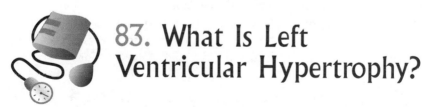

83. What Is Left Ventricular Hypertrophy?

Left ventricular hypertrophy (LVH) is thickening of the muscle of the left ventricle, which is the main pumping chamber of the heart. If the heart must continually work against increased pressure, it will, like any muscle, eventually thicken due to overwork. This "thickening" is called hypertrophy. The traditional analogy is the muscle in the blacksmith's arm, which, because of repeated pounding on the anvil, undergoes hypertrophy and becomes enlarged.

The best way of identifying LVH is to use an echocardiogram, which can visualize the size and configuration of the heart and the thickness of its muscular walls. In the routine evaluation of a patient with hypertension, an echocardiogram is not indicated, and most insurance companies will not pay for this type of imaging as part of the evaluation of the hypertensive patient unless a special reason exists. Furthermore, the physical examination, electrocardiogram, and chest X ray can often establish the diagnosis without the need for an echocardiogram.

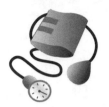

84. What Is a TIA and How Is It Treated?

A TIA (transient ischemic attack) is a transient decrease of blood supply to a portion of the brain. Often this event is the forerunner of a stroke. Indeed, a TIA is really a small stroke affecting speech and movement of extremities, or leading to temporary loss of vision in one eye. These spells usually last for less than 10 minutes, followed by complete recovery. TIAs probably occur when small thrombi (clots) break off from atherosclerotic plaques (damaged lining of arteries) in the neck or heart and temporarily block small arteries supplying the area of the brain that controls speech, movements of extremities, or vision.

A TIA (transient ischemic attack) is a transient decrease of blood supply to a portion of the brain.

Many, but not all, patients with TIAs are hypertensive. If they are, their blood pressures should be reduced gradually. Medical treatment includes aspirin, which prevents the formation of little thrombi, or coumadin, which is a stronger anticoagulant than aspirin. Sometimes it may be necessary to surgically remove a plaque (which is composed mainly of cholesterol and causes obstruction) in the carotid artery of the neck. Treating hypertension will reduce the risk of TIAs and major strokes.

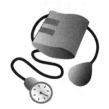

85. What Is a Stroke?

A stroke is a blockage or rupture of an artery in the brain, leading to destruction of the surrounding area of the brain. The result may be paralysis of one or more extremities, difficulty or inability to talk, or disturbed vision, depending upon which area of the brain is involved. Approximately 75% of all strokes occur in hypertensive persons, and treatment of high blood pressure will markedly reduce the risk of stroke.

A blockage of an artery in the brain may occur in several ways. For example, a brain artery may become blocked because of atherosclerosis and a clot formation within the artery. Alternatively, a cholesterol plaque may break off from a carotid artery in the neck or from the aorta and be carried by the bloodstream to an artery in the brain, which it obstructs. In addition, blood clots may form in the left atrium of the heart because of an irregularity of the heart rhythm known as atrial fibrillation.

> *A stroke is a blockage or rupture of an artery in the brain, leading to destruction of the surrounding area of the brain. Treatment of high blood pressure will markedly reduce the risk of stroke.*

Strokes may sometimes be prevented by surgery intended to prevent atherosclerotic plaques from reaching the brain. Your physician may recommend low-dose aspirin to prevent many types of stroke or coumadin (an anticoagulant) to prevent formation of blood clots in the heart and reduce the chance of an embolus (a clot) traveling to the brain, especially if you have experienced a heart attack or have atrial fibrillation.

86. What Is an Aneurysm? Can It Be Caused by Hypertension, and How Can It Be Detected and Treated?

An aneurysm is an abnormal enlargement or a bulge that balloons out in a portion of a blood vessel. It usually results from a weakness in the wall of an artery or the aorta (the largest artery in the body, which carries blood from the heart to arteries supplying blood throughout the body). Hypertension can cause aneurysms to enlarge and rupture; the ensuing hemorrhage can result in severe damage to surrounding tissue, which may prove fatal.

> *An aneurysm is an abnormal enlargement or a bulge that balloons out in a portion of a blood vessel. It usually results from a weakness in the wall of an artery or the aorta.*

The weakness of the wall of the artery or aorta usually results from atherosclerosis (hardening and damaging of the artery with deposits of cholesterol on the lining of the vessel). A small percentage of aneurysms are caused by traumatic injuries. Nearly 20% of aneurysms, however, are hereditary—the result of a genetic abnormality that weakens the vessel wall. These hereditary aneurysms can occur in the brain, where they are sometimes called "berry" aneurysms because they resemble a sac in the shape of a berry. They are sometimes associated with an abnormal constriction or narrowing of the aorta in the abdomen known as a coarctation. Coarctation can cause hypertension in the upper portion of the body, which increases the risk of hemorrhage from any coexisting aneurysms exposed to this increased blood pressure; pressure beyond the constriction in the lower portion of the body and in the legs is less than it is in the upper portion of the body (see Question 38). Alternatively, hereditary aneurysms may occur in the first part of the aorta as it leaves the heart. In these cases, they are frequently associated with an abnormality of the heart valve at the beginning of the aorta.

Occasionally an aneurysm may compress an artery supplying blood to a kidney. The impairment of the blood supply to the kidney may cause this organ to release an enzyme (renin), with subsequent generation of a hormone (angiotensin II) that can cause hypertension.

Approximately 75% of aortic aneurysms occur in the lower part of the abdomen and result from atherosclerosis. The prevalence of these aneurysms is greatest in the elderly, particularly those with hypertension, and their enlargements tend to grow with aging. Although they do not generally produce symptoms, they may become painful and tender, and cause pain in the abdomen and back as they enlarge. Sometimes these aneurysms may cause very severe pain because of a tear in the aorta, which may lead to a fatal hemorrhage if it ruptures. Often an abdominal aortic aneurysm is detected by the physician as a palpable, pulsatile, nontender mass in the abdomen; the diagnosis can be confirmed by imaging studies such as ultrasound, CAT scan, or MRI. The five-year risk of rupture with aneurysms less than 2 inches in diameter is 1% to 2%, whereas 20% to 40% of larger aneurysms will rupture within five years. Therefore, surgical repair with a graft is indicated for large aneurysms. Beta-blocking drugs are recommended for smaller aneurysms, because these agents reduce the strength of pulsations against the weakened aneurysmal wall and prevent further enlargement. Of course, it is crucial to reduce an elevated blood pressure to 135/85 mm Hg or less in case of abdominal aneurysm.

Aneurysms located elsewhere in the body may be identified by various imaging techniques and can be treated surgically, if indicated. Aneurysms in the brain may require a clipping procedure or a new surgical technique that places a coil in the aneurysm to obliterate it in order to prevent rupture and hemorrhage in the future.

Of paramount importance in avoiding possible rupture of an aneurysm is normalization of blood pressure with appropriate anti-hypertensive medication.

87. Do Hypertension, High Cholesterol, Obesity, and Diabetes Mellitus Often Go Together? How Do You Treat This "Deadly Quartet"?

The constellation of (1) hypertension, (2) abnormal blood fats, namely high LDL cholesterol (low-density lipoprotein, the "bad" cholesterol), low HDL (high-density lipoprotein, the "good" choles-terol), and high triglycerides (another "bad" fat), (3) central (upper body) obesity, and (4) insulin resis-tance (a decreased ability of insulin to metabolize and store sugar in muscle) and sometimes adult-onset diabetes mellitus has been correctly designated "the deadly quartet." Left untreated, this set of risk factors will often lead to severe vascular damage, resulting in heart attack, stroke, heart and kidney failure, damage to the eyes with visual impairment, weakening and rupture of blood vessels, impairment of blood flow to the lower extremities (some-times requiring amputation), and death.

The constellation of hypertension, abnormal blood fats, central (upper body) obesity, and insulin resistance/diabetes mellitus has been correctly designated "the deadly quartet."

Although the cause of insulin resistance remains poorly understood, this condition is known to be associated with development of obesity and may be aggravated by excess alcohol consumption. It is the underlying abnormality that leads to adult-onset diabetes mellitus, in which increased blood concentration of insulin occurs in an effort to compensate for the resistance to insulin metabolism of sugar. (In childhood diabetes, insulin levels in the blood are very low or absent.) Insulin resistance affects approximately 20% of the U.S. population and is almost always associ-ated with cardiovascular risk factors, including obesity, abnormal blood fats, hypertension, and salt sensitivity. Some believe that insulin may play a role in causing hypertension, but this is probably not the case.

There is no easy way of testing for insulin resistance, but the presence of other findings in the constellation of abnormalities mentioned earlier indirectly establishes its diagnosis. Treatment is directed at achieving the following goals:

- Reduction of blood pressure to less than 130/85 mm Hg
- Weight reduction, if indicated, by decreasing caloric intake with a low-cholesterol and low-saturated-fat diet, and increasing caloric expenditure with appropriate aerobic exercise
- Use of a low-salt diet—that is, no more than 6 grams (one teaspoonful of sodium chloride), equivalent to 2400 milligrams of sodium, per day
- Limitation of alcohol to only one or two drinks of spirits, wine, or beer per day
- Cessation of smoking
- Proper control of diabetes, if present

When antihypertensive medication is indicated, it should include an ACE or angiotensin II inhibitor, as these drug classes are particularly effective in preventing or minimizing the renal damage that is especially apt to occur in diabetics. For those patients requiring more than one drug, which is usually the case, diuretics (water pills) can prove valuable, as diabetics are frequently salt-sensitive and have fluid retention; atenolol (a beta blocker) is effective in such cases. Finally, low-dose aspirin is recommended when the blood pressure is controlled.

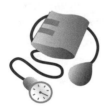

88. What Foods or Drinks Should I Avoid If I Have Hypertension?

Excess calories, fat, salt, and alcohol, and inadequate potassium may all play roles in the development and severity of hypertension.

If you have hypertension and are overweight, it is very important that you make a strong effort to reduce the number of calories in your diet. For most hypertensives who are overweight, weight loss is usually the most effective way of lowering blood pressure. Motivation is essential to dieting success, of course, and we recommend reduction of dietary fat to no more than 30% of your daily calories. This consideration is important: 1 gram (g) of fat equals 9 calories, whereas 1 g of protein or carbohydrate is equivalent to only 4 calories. For this reason, excess consumption of fat should be avoided to reduce and to maintain appropriate weight. Furthermore, limiting saturated fat and cholesterol in the diet is especially important if LDL (low-density lipoprotein, the "bad" cholesterol) is elevated or if HDL (high-density lipoprotein, the "good" cholesterol) is low, as this condition may hasten the development and progression of atherosclerosis (hardening of arteries). Reducing caloric intake also depends on reducing the amount of food consumed. Perhaps the most acceptable way of accomplishing this goal is to decrease portion size rather than to introduce a new, bland diet that the patient does not find palatable.

Curtailing the use of sodium chloride (table salt) is particularly important in salt-sensitive individuals—and an estimated 50% to 60% of essential hypertensives are salt-sensitive. These individuals may retain excess salt and water and develop hypertension. It is easy to limit excess salt in cooking and to avoid use of the salt shaker. Because 70% to 75% of salt is ordinarily consumed in processed foods, however, one should be constantly aware of the sodium content as indicated on the labels of various foods purchased in supermarkets or elsewhere (see Question 34). Note that some drinks and juices (such as Gatorade, tomato juice, and V8 juice) and some water supplies contain significant amounts of sodium. It is recommended that no more than 6 g of salt (about one teaspoonful), equivalent to 2400 milligrams of sodium, should be ingested daily.

Diets high in potassium (from liberal amounts of fruits and vegetables) appear to slowly lower blood pressure. Hence, low-potassium diets should be avoided. This mineral also protects against stroke, replaces some of the excess sodium in the body, and causes sodium to be excreted in the urine.

Of significant importance is the avoidance of excess alcohol in patients with essential hypertension. Excess alcohol consumption is reportedly responsible for elevated blood pressure in 7% to 10% of all hypertensive individuals. Men with hypertension should limit their intake to no more than two drinks (spirits, wine, or beer) per day, and women with hypertension should limit alcohol consumption to only one drink daily.

Excess ingestion of licorice is also known to induce hypertension. Licorice contains glycyrrhetinic acid, which causes sodium retention, potassium excretion, and development of hypertension. Licorice extracts are also present in chewing tobacco, so this substance should be avoided. In addition, certain food supplements (for example, those containing ephedrine or yohimbine) should be avoided, as they can constrict arterioles and cause hypertension. If caffeine-containing drinks cause you to experience excess elevations of blood pressure, it would be wise to switch to decaffeinated brands, especially if you have hypertension. Grapefruit can inhibit an enzyme that metabolizes some of the calcium-channel blockers, causing concentrations of the drugs to build up in the blood and exert a stronger effect in lowering blood pressure.

Finally, a word of caution about "health foods." Some supplements and herbal remedies may possibly interact with some antihypertensive medications. For example, ginseng may elevate blood pressure and ma huang may cause stroke, heart attack, and sudden death (see Questions 71, 73). You should always consult your physician before taking food supplements!

89. Why Is My Cholesterol Elevated? What Is the Desirable Level, and Should I Try to Lower It?

Your blood cholesterol may be elevated because of excess consumption of cholesterol and fat (some of which is converted to cholesterol). Note, however, that 75% of cholesterol is produced by the liver (a function that is determined by your genes). Lowering an elevated blood level of cholesterol through use of diet and medications may protect you from hardening of the arteries, heart attack, and stroke.

Total blood cholesterol for adults 30 years or older is considered normal if it is 200 mg or less. In adults 29 years or younger and in adolescents, this level should be 180 mg or less.

Total blood cholesterol for adults 30 years or older is considered normal if it is 200 milligrams (mg) or less. In adults 29 years or younger and in adolescents, this level should be 180 mg or less. Vegetarians usually have total cholesterol levels that are very low, often less than 150 mg.

Even a diet that contains very little cholesterol and fat may not normalize blood cholesterol if your liver inappropriately produces too much of this substance. Normally, increased consumption of cholesterol and saturated fat increases blood cholesterol, which is recognized by receptors (structures on liver cells that sense the blood level of cholesterol). Cholesterol in the blood attaches to these receptors, enters the liver cells, and then suppresses the production of cholesterol by the liver. If the number of these receptors is decreased, less cholesterol can enter the liver cells and the liver provides less suppression of cholesterol production. As a consequence, cholesterol in the blood becomes more elevated. Tragically, children in some families inherit few (if any) of these receptors, leading them to develop extremely high cholesterol levels; these children usually die at very young ages from heart attacks. Fortunately, this familial condition is extremely rare.

Cholesterol in the blood consists of three major components, which are carried in the blood as lipoproteins:

- Low-density lipoprotein (LDL)
- Very-low-density lipoprotein (VLDL)
- High-density lipoprotein (HDL)

The main lipoproteins in the blood are LDL and HDL. "Density" simply indicates the weight of these lipoproteins.

LDL is known as "bad" cholesterol, because it can lead to deposits of cholesterol (plaques) on the lining of blood vessels. Plaque formation can block arteries and cause heart attacks and strokes. The desirable level of LDL cholesterol is 130 mg or less. Slightly higher levels are acceptable if you have no other risk factors (that is, diabetes, cigarette smoking, evidence of coronary heart disease, hypertension, low HDL, or family history of premature heart attacks). If you are a man younger than 45 years old or a premenopausal woman, then slightly higher levels of LDL are of less concern. If you have evidence of heart disease, it is always desirable to keep the level of LDL cholesterol below 100 mg.

90. What Is the Story on "Good" and "Bad" Cholesterol and Triglycerides? Can Cholesterol Cause Hypertension?

HDL (high-density lipoprotein) is known as "good" cholesterol because it removes LDL (low-density lipoprotein), or "bad" cholesterol, from the arteries and carries it to the liver where it is excreted in the bile. Desirable levels of HDL are 45 milligrams (mg) or higher. In general, the higher the level of HDL, the lower the risk of heart disease. In addition, the ratio of total cholesterol to HDL appears to be one indicator for the chance of heart disease. An acceptable total cholesterol/HDL ratio is roughly 4.5 or less for men and 3.5 or less for women. LDL/HDL ratios are sometimes used to assess risk of heart disease, but are no more accurate than total cholesterol/HDL ratios in this respect.

Desirable levels of HDL are 45 mg or higher. An acceptable total cholesterol/HDL ratio is roughly 4.5 or less for men and 3.5 or less for women.

HDL may be increased by appropriate weight loss, aerobic exercise, some antihypertensive medications (alpha blockers), some drugs that are used to lower cholesterol and triglycerides (niacin, statins, and fibrates), consumption of modest amounts of alcohol, cessation of cigarette smoking, and estrogens. Conversely, HDL may be decreased by obesity, lack of exercise, some antihypertensive drugs (beta blockers), and smoking.

Very strong evidence shows that populations who consume lots of animal fats and dairy products have a high incidence of death from coronary heart disease, whereas those who consume diets high in fruits, vegetables, fish, and fat from olive oil have a much lower incidence of heart disease. Although cholesterol is essential for the production of cell membranes and hormones in the body, excessive amounts of LDL contribute to blood vessel and heart disease, particularly if some of this cholesterol is oxidized (that is, becomes combined with oxygen). Oxidized cholesterol is especially undesirable, as it is taken up by cells lining the arteries and forms plaques in these vessels. Antioxidants may reduce the formation of oxidized cholesterol, thereby protecting against hardening of the arteries (atherosclerosis). In addition, cholesterol-lowering drugs are used to prevent or minimize the damaging effect of excess cholesterol on arteries (see Question 92).

Triglycerides are another form of lipid (fat) that is mainly carried in the blood by VLDL (very-low-density lipoprotein). They may be elevated because of a genetic abnormality or because of an environmental influence (such as obesity, excess fat consumption, diabetes, or excess alcohol). Triglycerides become especially elevated shortly after you eat a fatty meal. Therefore, their concentration should be measured while the patient is fasting (fasting is not necessary when measuring total cholesterol, HDL, or LDL). **Elevated triglycerides appear to be a less important risk factor for coronary heart disease, but maintaining them at a level of 200 mg or less is still deemed desirable.** Very high levels of triglycerides (more than 500 mg) are considered a risk for developing pancreatitis (inflammation of the pancreas); pancreatitis has no relationship to hypertension, however.

Maintaining a normal blood concentration of cholesterol and triglycerides is important for preventing arterial damage, which can impair blood flow in the vessels of the heart, brain, and legs and result in heart attacks, stroke, and pain in the legs when walking. According to some reports, a 1% decline in a person's cholesterol level can reduce the risk of death from heart attacks by 2%. The presence of coronary heart disease mandates aggressive efforts to reduce LDL cholesterol and increase HDL cholesterol, if possible. Hypertension in the presence of an elevated LDL level compounds the problem, further accelerating vascular damage and therefore increasing the risk of heart attack and stroke. If lifestyle modifications do not normalize blood pressure and adequately reduce LDL cholesterol, then appropriate drug therapies are indicated. **An elevated cholesterol level does not cause hypertension, but it may produce hardening of the arteries, which can then result in systolic hypertension.**

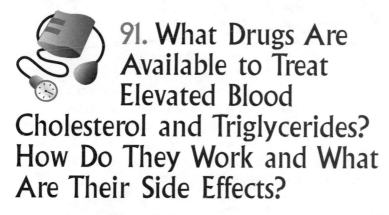

91. What Drugs Are Available to Treat Elevated Blood Cholesterol and Triglycerides? How Do They Work and What Are Their Side Effects?

Several classes of drugs are effective in lowering cholesterol and triglycerides, both of which are types of lipids (fats) found in the blood:

- Niacin (nicotinic acid)
- Bile acid-binding resins (Questran, Colestid)
- Fibrates (Lopid, Tricor)
- Statins (Lipitor, Baycol, Lescol, Mevacor, Pravachol, Zocor)

Table 12 describes their mechanisms of action and side effects.

Drugs that lower elevated blood concentrations of LDL cholesterol (low-density lipoprotein, also known as "bad" cholesterol) can cause regression of cholesterol plaques that partially obstruct arteries, improve blood flow, and reduce heart attacks and mortality. Therefore, it is extremely important to consider the use of drugs to lower blood cholesterol and triglycerides when dietary and lifestyle changes fail to reduce these lipid levels. Furthermore, it is critical to lower cholesterol and triglyceride levels in the presence of hypertension, as the combination of these two risk factors poses a far more serious health hazard than the presence of either risk factor by itself. The existence of other risk factors—such as coronary heart disease, diabetes, family history of premature death from heart attack or stroke, cigarette smoking, sedentary lifestyle, and obesity—may compound the problem and necessitate aggressive efforts to control both hypertension and lipid abnormalities.

As noted earlier, elevated cholesterol and triglyceride levels can have damaging effects on the lining of blood vessels. In contrast, high levels of HDL (high-density lipoprotein, also known as "good" cholesterol) may protect against such damage by removing and transporting deposits of cholesterol from plaques in the arteries to the liver. Thus a drug that effectively lowers both LDL cholesterol and triglycerides, while raising HDL cholesterol, would be especially desirable.

When lifestyle changes (weight reduction, exercise, restriction of fat to 30% of daily calories, and reduction of dietary cholesterol) fail to normalize elevated LDL and triglyceride levels, lipid-lowering drugs should be considered. In general, the higher the levels of LDL and triglycerides and the greater the number of risk factors, the more aggressive the effort to combat any correctable conditions should be. The important protective role played by elevated HDL levels must also be considered. Women generally have higher levels of HDL than men do, and often these levels are markedly elevated and mainly account for the elevation of total cholesterol. An elevated total cholesterol level that results mainly from an elevated HDL level obviously requires no treatment.

Desirable levels of total cholesterol, LDL, HDL, and triglycerides were discussed in Question 90. Table 12 lists the various drugs available to treat any lipid abnormalities. All of these drugs can reduce the incidence of nonfatal heart attacks as well as mortality from heart attacks. Unfortunately, the medications may cause undesirable side effects, so your physician may not use them with mild lipid abnormalities that can be corrected by lifestyle changes.

When use of these drugs becomes necessary, your physician will probably suggest starting with a statin. Statins work by inhibiting the enzyme that produces cholesterol, so they are very effective in lowering LDL. In addition, they are moderately effective in lowering triglycerides and may sometimes slightly increase HDL. The statins are generally better tolerated than other lipid-lowering drugs are. Although side effects are infrequent and usually not severe with these agents, liver enzymes may become elevated indicating some liver toxicity. This effect is typically mild and requires no change in treatment. If the enzyme changes are pronounced, however, it may be necessary to discontinue medication; elevated enzyme levels almost invariably return to normal after use of a statin ends. Very rarely, muscle pains with severe muscle damage may occur and be accompanied by kidney failure. The combination of a statin and a fibrate can increase the risk of severe muscle damage, though it remains a rare occurrence.

Niacin (for example, Niaspan) can lower both LDL and triglyceride levels, and it usually increases HDL levels very significantly. The mechanism of action that produces these effects remains unknown. Flushing is

Table 12. *Medications Used to Lower LDL Cholesterol and Triglycerides and to Increase HDL Cholesterol*

Drug	Mechanism of Action	Effects on			Side Effects
		LDL	Triglycerides	HDL	
Niacin (Niaspan)	Unknown	↓	↓	↑↑	Flushing, itching, fatigue, blurred vision, ↑ blood sugar, indigestion, peptic ulcer flare-up, liver inflammation.
Resins (Questran, Colestid)	Bind with bile acids and prevent reabsorption of cholesterol from intestine	↓	0	0	Constipation, indigestion, nausea
Fibrates (Lopid, Tricor)	Uncertain but decreases production of triglycerides by liver and decreases VLDL, which carries triglycerides in blood	↑↓	↓↓	↑↑	Indigestion, rash. May increase effectiveness of anticoagulants and drugs that lower blood sugar. May interact with statins and cause muscle damage, gallstones, and kidney failure.
Statins (Lipitor, Baycol, Lescol, Mevacor, Pravachol, Zocor)	Inhibit HMG-CoA reductase, decrease production of cholesterol by the liver, and increase its removal from the blood	↓↓	↓	(↑)	Increased liver enzymes, rash, itching, headache, muscle pains, and damage accompanied by kidney failure. May interact with fibrates and cause muscle damage.

Key: ↑ increase; ↑↑ considerable increase; (↑) may sometimes increase slightly; ↓ decrease; ↓↓ considerable decrease; 0 no change; ↑↓ variable effects.

Note: Regular consumption of Benecol may lower LDL cholesterol by up to 14% in persons with elevated cholesterol. This margarine-like compound contains a plant substance, sitostanol, which inhibits cholesterol absorption from the intestine with no apparent side effects. It is relatively low in calories and sodium and may be a good substitute for butter; however, you should consult your physician before using it during pregnancy.

This table may be helpful for you to discuss with your physician.

the most common and annoying side effect, but can often be minimized or prevented by the concomitant use of aspirin.

Resins (Questran or Colestid) bind with bile acids, which contain cholesterol, and increase the elimination of cholesterol in the stool. Some patients find them unpalatable, and many complain of constipation and indigestion. Although resins are fairly effective in reducing LDL cholesterol, they have no effect on triglycerides or HDL. Other medications should be taken at least two hours before consumption of a resin, as the resin may interfere with the other drugs' absorption.

Fibrates (Lopid and Tricor) are very effective in lowering triglycerides and increasing HDL, but have variable effect on LDL. Any increase or decrease in LDL level is generally slight, if it occurs. The precise mechanism of action for the fibrates remains to be elucidated, although the drugs are known to decrease the liver's production of triglycerides. These drugs may potentiate both the effect of anticoagulants (blood thinners) and the effect of some drugs used to lower blood sugar.

Of the drugs used to control lipid abnormalities, the statins appear most suitable for lowering LDL cholesterol levels; they also sometimes lower triglyceride levels. If side effects prevent continuing use of the statins, then niacin and the resins are good choices. For marked elevations of triglycerides, the fibrates are most effective in normalizing the lipid concentrations; these drugs have little effect on LDL levels, however. The choice of the appropriate drug and its dosage, monitoring of liver enzymes, recognition of side effects, and avoidance of drug interactions that could cause harm are the responsibility of the physician.

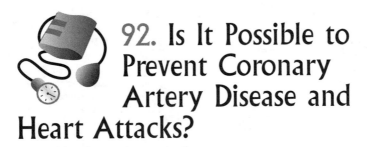

92. Is It Possible to Prevent Coronary Artery Disease and Heart Attacks?

It is very possible to prevent heart disease. The major risk factors for coronary artery disease are hypertension, high blood cholesterol, and cigarette smoking. All of these conditions can contribute to hardening of the arteries (atherosclerosis) and subsequent impairment of blood flow to the heart, which can in turn lead to angina (chest pain or pressure sensation) and heart attack. Well-conducted clinical trials have confirmed that controlling high blood pressure, controlling high cholesterol, and stopping cigarette smoking markedly reduce a person's risk of coronary heart disease and heart attack. The highest incidences of heart attack occur in nations whose populations consume the highest amounts of dairy products, saturated fats, and cholesterol. Regular aerobic exercise (see Question 46), if not contraindicated, may lower elevated blood pressure, aid in maintaining proper weight, elevate "good" cholesterol, lower "bad" cholesterol, and thus prevent or minimize coronary artery disease. In addition, some preliminary evidence suggests that elevations of homocysteine in the blood may cause atherosclerosis; therefore, it seems prudent to reduce significantly high homocysteine levels (see Question 94).

Diabetes mellitus is also a major risk factor for atherosclerosis and coronary heart disease. Unfortunately, tight control of the blood sugar of diabetics does not appear to reduce this risk, although this practice does lessen the risk of kidney, nerve, and eye complications. If you have diabetes, it is very important that you keep your blood pressure and cholesterol under good control and that you do not smoke cigarettes.

93. If I Am Very Old, Do I Need Treatment for Hypertension or High Cholesterol?

A recent review of the numerous trials that included elderly patients (older than 65 years) revealed that **the benefits of antihypertensive therapy are even greater for older patients than they are for younger patients.** This finding probably reflects the fact that older patients are at greater risk for cardiovascular disease than younger patients—hence the benefits from treatment are correspondingly greater. Older patients who receive treatment for their high blood pressure have fewer strokes, fewer heart attacks, and less congestive heart failure than do elderly patients with untreated hypertension. This relationship holds true for patients up to and including 85 years of age. We have no reason to believe that it will not apply to patients older than this, though the treatment trials to date have not included enough patients older than age 85 to draw any definite conclusions.

The benefits of treating elevated "bad" cholesterol (LDL—low-density lipoprotein) with medication in elderly men, especially in those with low levels of "good" cholesterol (HDL—high-density lipoprotein), are fairly well established. On the other hand, less evidence has been gathered to prove beneficial effects from treating elevated "bad" cholesterol in women at any age. Most women have relatively high levels of "good" cholesterol in their blood, which protects them from cardiovascular disease. If a woman has a pronounced elevation of "bad" cholesterol and a low level of "good" cholesterol, however, it seems reasonable to reduce the "bad" cholesterol with appropriate medication. Reduction of significantly elevated levels of triglycerides in the blood is desirable in both genders. Lifestyle changes are, of course, always recommended when indicated.

The benefits of treating elevated LDL levels with medication in elderly men, especially in those with low HDL levels, are fairly well established. Less evidence has been gathered to prove beneficial effects from treating elevated "bad" (LDL) cholesterol in women at any age.

94. What Is Homocysteine? Does It Have Harmful Effects and What Should I Do If I Have an Excess Amount?

Homocysteine is an amino acid (a substance used by the body to manufacture proteins) that is normally present in your blood. Some concern has arisen that elevated levels of homocysteine in the blood are correlated with damage to blood vessels, development of hardening of the arteries (atherosclerosis), and risk of heart attack and stroke. Elevations of homocysteine in the blood result in excessive amounts of homocysteine in the urine (homocysteinuria). Children with homocysteinuria due to a hereditary abnormality develop hardening of the arteries as frequently as do older adults. Thus it appears that elevated homocysteine levels in the blood accelerate the development of atherosclerosis.

Homocysteine is an amino acid that is normally present in your blood. Some concern has arisen that elevated levels of homocysteine in the blood are correlated with damage to blood vessels, development of hardening of the arteries, and risk of heart attack and stroke.

Approximately 10% of all people have a defective version of the enzyme that ordinarily clears homocysteine from the blood. Such a defect enables abnormally high amounts of homocysteine to become concentrated in the blood. However, the main reason for homocysteine elevations is inadequate consumption of folic acid, vitamin B$_6$, and vitamin B$_{12}$, all of which are found in vegetables (especially lima beans and broccoli). Low levels of folic acid in the blood have been linked to high levels of homocysteine and increased risk of heart disease. An estimated 40% of Americans consume inadequate amounts of folic acid.

Because of the risk and complications of hardening of the arteries (including heart attacks, strokes, and blood vessel disease), **it is recommended that folic acid be taken daily if the homocysteine level in the blood is elevated or the folic acid level is abnormally low.** The presence of hypertension could aggravate the complications of atherosclerosis if homocysteine is elevated in the blood. Nevertheless, homocysteine in the blood is very rarely measured, as its role in causing hardening of the arteries remains controversial.

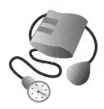

95. Are High Cholesterol and High Blood Pressure Related?

High blood pressure and high blood cholesterol are both recognized as important risk factors for heart disease, arterial disease, and stroke, but they act independently of each other. A person can have high blood pressure without high cholesterol, and vice versa. Certainly patients with high blood cholesterol should be checked for hypertension, and individuals with hypertension should be checked for high blood cholesterol, because the combination of the two conditions represents a powerful risk factor for heart disease and stroke. If the high blood cholesterol results in hardening of the arteries (atherosclerosis) and hence decreased elasticity of the aorta and large arteries, systolic blood pressure would increase as well.

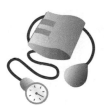

96. What Are Antioxidants and Should I Be Taking Them?

The excitement and interest voiced by both the public and the medical profession in the possible benefits of antioxidants in the prevention of a variety of chronic diseases have been enormous. The antioxidants that have been most extensively evaluated for their therapeutic effects are vitamin E (tocopherol), vitamin C (ascorbic acid), beta-carotene (which is converted to vitamin A in the body), and many other carotenoids.

The antioxidants that have been most extensively evaluated for their therapeutic effects are vitamin E (tocopherol), vitamin C (ascorbic acid), beta-carotene (which is converted to vitamin A in the body), and many other carotenoids.

The main sources of antioxidants are fruits and vegetables, although tea is also a notable source. Although the National Cancer Institute and the National Research Council recommend that we eat five servings of both fruits and vegetables each day for optimal health, in reality only a very small percentage of Americans consume these amounts.

Antioxidants act as "scavengers" or "traps" of certain harmful chemicals, thereby preventing or minimizing the harmful effects of oxidation by-products of normal body metabolism. These harmful by-products consist of "free radicals"—unstable, toxic chemical agents. Some evidence indicates that these free radicals may cause extensive damage to DNA, proteins, carbohydrates, and lipids in cells and tissues; increase cell division; and eventually lead to injury and clogging of arteries and to development of cancer. Cigarette smoking and ultraviolet radiation are environmental factors that can promote the formation of free radicals.

Strong evidence shows that groups who consume low amounts of fruits and vegetables have high rates of heart disease and cancer (particularly of the lung, larynx, oral cavity, esophagus, stomach, colon, rectum, urinary bladder, pancreas, cervix, and ovary; breast cancer incidence is only modestly increased in this population). Furthermore, some have speculated that antioxidants may not only prevent or retard progression of artery and heart disease and many types of cancer, but also oppose the development of immune system and neurological disorders, brain dysfunction, cataracts, and degenerative, aging-related diseases. As yet, however, the value of antioxidants in the treatment or prevention of various diseases remains to be established.

In two large studies of persons consuming large doses (100 international units [IU] or more) of vitamin E, this consumption reduced development of coronary artery heart disease by 50%; no such benefit was derived from consuming large doses of vitamin C. A recent study (reported in the *New England Journal of Medicine*) of patients at risk for cardiovascular disease found no therapeutic benefit after subjects consumed large amounts of vitamin E for five years.

Vitamin E appears to reduce the normal tendency for platelets (small, cell-like structures in the blood) to aggregate and form clots.

On the other hand, large doses of vitamin C have been reported to modestly lower blood cholesterol and blood pressure, although these findings are not a compelling reason to use vitamin C supplements. Far more effective ways of lowering blood cholesterol exist, and any effect on blood pressure from vitamin C consumption is minimal, if it occurs at all. Furthermore, large or megadoses (1000 milligrams or more daily) of vitamin C can cause an acid urine with a tendency toward kidney stone formation.

The effects of beta-carotene and other carotenoids have been less extensively studied, and their effectiveness as antioxidants remains unclear. No evidence shows that they have any effect on blood pressure or blood levels of cholesterol. The carotenoids' ability to prevent coronary artery damage, heart disease, and cancer remains under investigation.

It seems reasonable for individuals to consider taking vitamin E for its possible ability to reduce damage to arteries and mortality from heart attack, even though this protective effect remains unproved. The recommended dose of vitamin E is 400 IU daily; vitamin E has no side effects, even when consumed as megadoses. (Bottles containing vitamin E should be placed in the refrigerator after they are opened.)

The authors are "believers" in this supplementation. We take 400 IU of vitamin E daily, even though its therapeutic value has not been established!

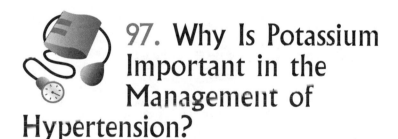

97. Why Is Potassium Important in the Management of Hypertension?

Increasing attention has focused on the importance of dietary potassium in reducing elevated blood pressure. A recent article in the prestigious *New England Journal of Medicine* emphasized that the DASH (Dietary Approaches to Stop Hypertension) diet, which contains lots of fruits and vegetables (a rich source of potassium) and also is low in fat, can lower both systolic and diastolic blood pressure. This diet consists of grains, fruits, vegetables, low-fat or nonfat dairy foods, meats, poultry, fish, nuts, seeds, and legumes (Table 13).

In one study, the DASH diet reduced fat consumption to approximately 27% of the total diet, down from the average fat intake

Table 13. *The DASH Diet (Based on about 2000 calories per Day)*

Food Group	Daily Servings	Serving Sizes	Examples	Significance to the DASH Diet
Grains, grain products	7–8	1 slice bread ½ cup dry cereal ½ cup cooked rice, pasta, or cereal	Whole-wheat bread, English muffin, pita bread, bagel, cereals, grits, oatmeal	Major sources of energy and fiber
Vegetables	4–5	1 cup raw, leafy vegetable ½ cup cooked vegetable 6 oz vegetable juice	Tomatoes, potatoes, carrots, peas, squash, broccoli, turnip greens, collards, kale, spinach, artichokes, beans, sweet potatoes	Rich sources of potassium, magnesium, and fiber
Fruits	4–5	6 oz fruit juice 1 medium fruit ¼ cup dried fruit ½ cup fresh, frozen, or canned fruit	Apricots, bananas, dates, oranges, grapefruit, mangoes, melons, peaches, pineapples, prunes, raisins, strawberries, tangerines	Important sources of potassium, magnesium, and fiber
Low-fat or nonfat dairy foods	2–3	8 oz milk 1 cup yogurt 1½ oz cheese	Skim or 1% milk, skim or low-fat buttermilk, nonfat or low-fat yogurt, part-skim mozzarella cheese, nonfat cheese	Major sources of calcium and protein
Meats, poultry, fish	2 or less	3 oz cooked meats, poultry, or fish	Select only lean meat; trim away visible fats; broil, roast, or boil instead of frying; remove skin from poultry	Rich sources of protein and magnesium
Nuts, seeds, legumes	4–5 per week	1½ oz or ⅓ cup nuts ½ oz or 2 tablespoons seeds ½ cup cooked legumes	Almonds, filberts, mixed nuts, peanuts, walnuts, sunflower seeds, kidney beans, lentils	Rich sources of energy, magnesium, potassium, protein, and fiber

Note: The DASH diet is rich in fruits, vegetables, and low-fat dairy foods and low in cholesterol, total fat, and saturated fat. It is high in fiber, potassium, calcium, and magnesium, and moderately high in protein.

Source: Dietary approaches to stop hypertension (DASH). The sixth report of the Joint National Committee. November 1997.

of 37%. After eight weeks on this diet, hypertensive patients experienced reductions in their systolic and diastolic pressures of 11.4 and 5.5 mm Hg, respectively. This decline occurred without change in alcohol or salt consumption, or weight loss, any of which by itself might have reduced blood pressure. The DASH diet also lowered the blood pressure of subjects with borderline elevations, suggesting that it may be helpful in preventing hypertension.

Potassium, a mineral similar to sodium, apparently replaces and eliminates excess sodium from body tissues, which reduces blood pressure in humans and animals with salt-sensitive hypertension. Potassium also dilates blood vessels. It is noteworthy that such supplements lower blood pressure more dramatically in hypertensive individuals than they do in nonhypertensive subjects; this antihypertensive effect on systolic and diastolic blood pressures is more pronounced in subjects on a high-salt diet.

> *Potassium apparently replaces and eliminates excess sodium from body tissues, which reduces blood pressure in humans and animals with salt-sensitive hypertension.*

An earlier report in the *New England Journal of Medicine* revealed that diets high in potassium may protect against stroke. An increase in daily potassium intake of even one serving of fresh fruits or vegetables was associated with a 40% reduction in the risk of stroke! The authors of this report also noted that protection from stroke was not necessarily related to the level of the blood pressure. The protective effect of fruits and vegetables against strokes in men was confirmed recently in a report appearing in another prestigious journal, the *Journal of the American Medical Association*.

Of seminal interest is the extraordinary finding reported about 16 years ago by Dr. Louis Tobian and his associates—namely, that dietary potassium could almost totally prevent stroke in stroke-prone rats with hypertension and in salt-induced hypertensive rats. In contrast, a very high percentage of rats with similar levels of hypertension but receiving a low-potassium diet died from strokes. The explanation of how potassium prevents strokes is not clear. A number of hypotheses have been proposed, but the mechanism of protection remains elusive and none of the hypotheses has been proven as yet.

Our own experimental research on salt-sensitive rats has shed some new light on this subject and probably best explains how potassium prevents strokes and kidney damage in the rat model. In our investigations, consumption of a liberal amount of dietary potassium considerably reduced blood pressure and markedly improved the circulation of the brain and kidney. This return of the circulation toward the normal pattern appears to prevent strokes and minimize damage to the kidneys. Similar changes might occur in humans with salt-sensitive hypertension; confirming this notion, however, requires further studies. The bottom line is that consumption of foods rich in potassium, especially fruits and vegetables, may both lower blood pressure and reduce the occurrence of stroke. It is also conceivable that a potassium-rich diet may minimize the development of hypertension in individuals with borderline elevations of blood pressure.

Some experimental studies suggest that an increase in potassium in the blood may inhibit formation of harmful free radicals (metabolic oxidation products), inhibit undesirable smooth muscle growth in the arteries, and prevent formation of blood clots. These changes would tend to prevent hardening of the arteries (atherosclerosis) and protect against cardiovascular disease. As yet, all of these effects remain theoretical possibilities that require further studies to prove them.

Greater consumption of foods rich in potassium appears to have no harmful effects in normal subjects. In some individuals with kidney disease or in patients taking antihypertensive drugs that retain potassium (such as ACE inhibitors and potassium-sparing diuretics), intake of large amounts of potassium through diet, medications, or salt substitutes may cause dangerous elevations of potassium in the blood that can create a serious disturbance in heart rhythm.

Nevertheless, fruits and vegetables should be consumed very frequently by most people. This recommendation is especially important for African Americans, who tend to eat relatively small amounts of fruits and vegetables and have a particularly high occurrence of hypertension, stroke, and kidney failure.

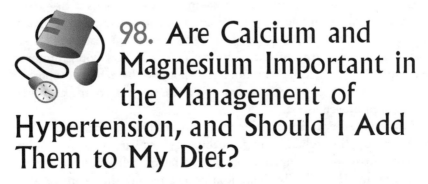

98. Are Calcium and Magnesium Important in the Management of Hypertension, and Should I Add Them to My Diet?

Calcium is important in many bodily functions, including muscle contraction, bone formation, blood clotting, hormone and enzyme activity, and functioning of cell membranes. Some reports indicate that a low calcium intake is responsible for elevations in blood pressure and that increasing dietary calcium may lower blood pressure. Analysis of a large number of studies suggests that adding 1000 to 2000 milligrams (mg) per day of calcium to the diet of patients on moderate calcium intake results in a small decrease in systolic blood pressure. Calcium appears to lower blood pressure in some persons with salt-sensitive hypertension by promoting elimination of salt and water. To date, however, the results of increasing dietary calcium or using calcium supplements to lower blood pressure have been disappointing. Consequently, use of calcium to lower blood pressure is not advised.

To date, the results of increasing dietary calcium or using calcium supplements to lower blood pressure have been disappointing. Consequently, use of calcium to lower blood pressure is not advised.

Adequate consumption of calcium is important in the prevention of osteoporosis (a condition in which bones lose calcium, which makes them brittle and easy to fracture). Bone density can be measured radiographically to determine the degree of osteoporosis present.

Although it is recommended that individuals younger than 65 years of age consume 1000 mg and those older than age 65 consume 1500 mg of calcium daily, this goal is rarely achieved by diet alone. Fat-free and low-fat dairy products (milk, cheese, yogurt), canned fish with bones, some vegetables (navy beans, turnips, broccoli), and many foods that are fortified with calcium (and often vitamin D) are excellent and healthy sources of this mineral. Calcium absorption from the intestine is enhanced by vitamin D, which should also be added to the diet if the patient shows evidence of osteoporosis. If you take a multivitamin tablet on a daily basis, you should choose supplemental calcium that is *not* fortified with vitamin D, because excess vitamin D can be toxic. Supplemental calcium is available in a variety of tablets; in addition, antacids such as Rolaids and Tums contain approximately 500 mg per tablet and can be used as a source of calcium. It is preferable to use a calcium citrate supplement that does not require acid in the stomach for optimal absorption; this type of pill can be taken any time during the day.

Some people have wondered whether the calcium antagonists (calcium-channel blockers) used to lower blood pressure could interfere with bodily functions other than dilating arteries, slowing heart rate, and exerting beneficial effects on heart muscle function. In fact, these drugs do not significantly alter function elsewhere in the body. In particular, calcium antagonists do not affect calcium metabolism in bone or influence the development or treatment of osteoporosis. Long-acting thiazide diuretics (water pills) used to lower blood pressure, on the other hand, cause retention of calcium by the body, which would tend to benefit patients with osteoporosis. Loop diuretics have the opposite effect, promoting loss of calcium from the body.

One word of caution: taking megadoses (very large amounts) of calcium and vitamin D can be very toxic and result in kidney stones and damage to the kidneys. More is not necessarily better!

Magnesium is even less effective in lowering blood pressure than is calcium. No good evidence suggests that this mineral can decrease blood pressure, so no reason exists to give magnesium supplements unless the patient has a magnesium deficit. Note, however, that magnesium sulfate given intravenously may help prevent convulsive seizures in patients with severe hypertension and eclampsia in pregnant women. Magnesium plays an important role in the action of enzymes, cell membrane function, and protein metabolism, and it may block calcium channels. It is recommended that men and women consume 350 mg/day and 265 mg/day of magnesium, respectively. Good sources of magnesium include green leafy vegetables, whole grains, meats, poultry, fish, seeds, nuts, and water.

A healthy diet should contain the recommended amounts of calcium and magnesium, but administration of these minerals does not offer a significant benefit in the treatment of hypertension.

99. What Causes Low Blood Pressure and Is It Harmful? What Are the Symptoms of Low Blood Pressure, in Case My Medication Is Excessive?

In general, it can be said that "the lower the blood pressure, the better"—as long as the individual does not have any symptoms of low blood pressure (see Question 77). This statement is true because the risks of heart attack and stroke are lower when blood pressure remains at a relatively low level.

For many years, a systolic blood pressure of 140 mm Hg and a diastolic pressure of 90 mm Hg were considered normal. Elevations above these levels were designated as hypertension, and they were associated with an increased chance of stroke, heart attack, heart and kidney failure, and impaired vision. It is true that the frequency of these complications increases as blood pressure becomes more elevated. More recently, however, physicians have recognized that the chance of these complications progressively decreases as blood pressure becomes significantly lower than 140/90 mm Hg. Optimal blood pressure levels appear to be about 120/80 mm Hg. Many normal young women, especially those who are underweight and have thin arms, have blood pressures of 90/60 mm Hg or slightly less, without any symptoms suggesting that their pressures are too low. It is also normal for blood pressure in the first and especially the second trimesters of pregnancy to decrease below the corresponding levels of nonpregnant women.

Abnormally low blood pressure, known as hypotension, may result when a person stands (postural hypotension) if some defect in sympathetic nerve activity causes an impairment of constriction of blood vessels; such a nerve-related defect may occur in some diseases of the nervous system, diabetes, and certain adrenal gland tumors. Other causes of hypotension include severe dehydration, blood loss, and allergic reactions. Various types of heart disease (especially those causing rate and rhythm disturbances) can also cause a sudden, momentary drop in blood pressure. A particularly common type of sudden drop in blood pressure, which occurs more frequently in young individuals, is due to a vasovagal reflex (a simple faint). This reflex of the nervous system dilates blood vessels and slows the heart rate, thereby leading to a dramatic decline in blood pressure. This condition may result from sudden anxiety and fear or from an emotionally upsetting experience, such as the sight of blood. It does not result from a disease or disability—even a Marine may experience the vasovagal reflex! In addition, overmedication with drugs that lower blood pressure can cause hypotension, with the blood pressure drop being particularly apt to occur when the patient is in the standing position.

Abnormally low blood pressure, known as hypotension, may result when a person stands (postural hypotension) if some defect in sympathetic nerve activity causes an impairment of constriction of blood vessels. Hypotension may also result from severe dehydration, blood loss, allergic reactions, heart disease, vasovagal reflex, or overmedication with blood-pressure-lowering drugs.

Hypotension is usually accompanied by lightheadedness, faintness, unsteadiness, and a rapid heart beat. In some instances, mental confusion, impaired vision, and temporary loss of consciousness may occur, which, of course, may result in a fall and serious injury. Chronic fatigue is not a symptom of hypotension.

Postural hypotension is more apt to occur in elderly and frail persons, especially if they are inactive or bedridden. For this reason, elderly patients are often started on lower doses of antihypertensive drugs than are younger and more robust individuals. It is important that older patients on antihypertensive medications take extra time in getting out of bed during the night and when arising in the morning. Sitting on the side of the bed for a minute or two and then holding onto something stable (such as a chair or table) may permit these individuals' vascular systems and blood pressures to better adjust to the change in posture, thereby preventing symptoms of hypotension and loss of consciousness.

A special warning should be given to all patients who take alpha-blocking drugs (such as Minipress, Hytrin, or Cardura), as these medications block the sympathetic nerves from causing blood vessel constriction. This constriction normally occurs on standing and prevents blood from pooling in the legs due to the effect of gravity. **A small percentage of patients will experience a marked drop in blood pressure when they stand up after taking their first dose of an alpha blocker** (see Question 66). The good news is that marked postural hypotension does not continue with subsequent use of these drugs.

Other commonly used antihypertensive drugs typically do not cause a marked, sudden drop in blood pressure. The ability of some short-acting calcium-channel blockers (such as Procardia) to cause a rapid drop in blood pressure is undesirable and potentially dangerous, as the resulting hypotension can significantly decrease the blood supply to the heart and brain and possibly produce a heart attack or stroke. For this reason, short-acting calcium-channel blockers are no longer used to treat hypertension.

Some antihypertensive drugs reduce blood pressure more rapidly than others do. If you take antihypertensive drugs and experience lightheadedness or feel you are going to faint, you should immediately sit or (preferably) lie down, as this position should reduce the effect of postural hypotension and improve the circulation to the brain. To document whether your lightheadedness or faint feeling is due to postural hypotension caused by your antihypertensive medication, it is essential to determine whether a pronounced drop in blood pressure occurs when you change from a recumbent or seated position to a standing position. Consult your physician immediately if you experience symptoms of hypotension so that your medication can be adjusted, if necessary.

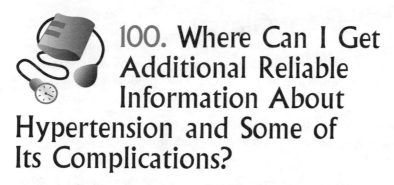

100. Where Can I Get Additional Reliable Information About Hypertension and Some of Its Complications?

American Heart Association
7272 Greenville Avenue
Dallas, TX 75231-4596
Web site:
www.amhrt.org
www.mediconsult.com
www.heartinfo.org

American Society of Hypertension
515 Madison Avenue,
Suite 1212
New York, NY 10022
Telephone: 212-644-0650
Web site:
www.ash-us.org

Mayo Clinic Health Oasis
Web site:
www.mayohealth.org

National Heart, Lung, and Blood Institute
P.O. Box 30105
Bethesda, MD 20824-0105
Recorded information:
800-575-9355
Web site:
www.nhlbi.nih.gov

National Hypertension Association
324 East 30th Street
New York, NY 10016
Telephone: 212-889-3557
Web site:
www.nathypertension.org

National Kidney Foundation
30 East 33rd Street
New York, NY 10016
Telephone: 800-622-9010
Web site:
www.kidney.org

National Stroke Association
96 Inverness Drive East, Suite 1
Englewood, CO 80112-5112
Telephone: 1-800-787-6537
Web site:
www.stroke.org

Glossary

ACE inhibitor—A drug that lowers blood pressure by inhibiting the angiotensin-converting enzyme (ACE) from producing angiotensin, which constricts arteries and arterioles and elevates blood pressure.

Acromegaly—An endocrine disease causing enlargement of parts of the skeleton due to oversecretion of growth hormone by the pituitary gland.

Adrenaline—A hormone from the adrenal gland that can increase the rate and pumping action of the heart, constrict some arterioles, and dilate other arterioles.

Aerobic exercise—Activity requiring motion that increases oxygen consumption, such as walking, running, bicycling, swimming, and other sports activities.

Alcohol dehydrogenase—An enzyme in the digestive tract that metabolizes alcohol.

Aldosterone—A hormone from the adrenal gland that causes the kidney to retain sodium and excrete potassium.

Alpha-adrenergic blocker—A drug that blocks noradrenaline (a hormone that constricts arterioles) from stimulating receptors on arterioles, thereby causing arterioles to dilate and lowering blood pressure.

Alpha-adrenergic receptors—"Targets" on various cells that, when stimulated by noradrenaline (or similar substances), cause a number of responses including constriction of arteries and arterioles, which in turn causes hypertension.

Anaerobic exercise—Activity requiring minimal motion without much increase in intake of oxygen, such as weightlifting.

Aneroid sphygmomanometer—A sphygmomanometer that measures blood pressure on a dial, and which depends on displacement of a spring rather than a mercury column. This device's accuracy should be compared periodically with results of a mercury sphygmomanometer, as the latter is the most reliable method for measuring blood pressure.

Aneurysm—A small or large dilatation—that is, a "ballooning out"—in the wall of an artery due to a weakness in the arterial wall.

Angina pectoris—A heaviness, pressure, squeezing sensation, or pain in the chest due to insufficient blood supply to the heart, usually brought on by exertion or emotional upset and relieved by rest.

Angioplasty—A technique using a catheter with a balloon that can be inflated to expand an artery.

Angiotensin—A substance in the blood (formed by renin) that is a powerful constrictor of arteries and arterioles.

Anticoagulant—Any substance that prevents blood from coagulating (clotting).

Antihypertensive medications—Drugs that lower elevated blood pressure.

Antioxidants—Substances that prevent the harmful oxidation effects of certain chemicals in the body that may cause hardening of the arteries and cancer.

Aorta—The largest artery in the body, which carries oxygenated blood pumped from the left muscular chamber of the heart, extends through the chest and abdomen, and branches into arteries supplying blood to the entire body.

Apnea—A transient cessation of breathing.

Arrhythmia—Abnormal rhythm or rate of the heart.

Arteries—The vessels that carry blood from the aorta to all parts of the body and end in arterioles, which then are connected to the capillaries.

Arterioles--The smallest arteries that carry blood from larger arteries to capillaries, which in turn supply tissues with blood. Arterioles have smooth muscle in their walls that permits constriction or dilation and thus can raise or lower blood pressure.

Arteriosclerosis—"Hardening" of an artery due to thickness of the wall, which causes a loss of elasticity.

Atherosclerosis—"Hardening" of an artery with deposits of cholesterol and blood cells on the inner lining of the artery, accompanied by the formation of plaques that can partially or totally impede blood flow.

Atrial fibrillation—Irregular rapid movements of the atrial muscles without normal contraction to expel blood from the two small chambers of the heart into the ventricles.

Atrium—One of a pair of small chambers of the heart, which receive blood from veins and expel it into the ventricles, the pumping chambers of the heart.

Beta-adrenergic blocker—A drug that lowers blood pressure mainly by blocking beta receptors on the heart, which slows the heart rate, and kidney, thereby preventing release of renin from the kidneys and inhibiting the production of a substance (angiotensin II) that constricts arterioles.

Beta-adrenergic receptors—"Targets" on various cells that, when stimulated by adrenaline and noradrenaline (or similar substances), cause a number of responses including those related to an increased rate and strength of heart muscle contraction, which can increase blood pressure.

Biofeedback—A technique designed to aid an individual to sense or feel a change in bodily function (e.g., heart rate or blood pressure), which permits the individual to lower his or her blood pressure and heart rate by control of mental and bodily function (e.g., increased relaxation).

Blood pressure—The pressure exerted by the blood against the walls of the arteries.

Body mass index—A measure of ideal and excessive weight; a weight-to-height index calculated by dividing weight in kilograms by the square of height in meters.

Brand-name drugs—Drugs named by the manufacturing pharmaceutical company and protected by a patent; they are more expensive than generic drugs but no more effective.

Bruit—A sound or murmur usually heard near or over a narrowed artery and occurring with each heart beat.

Calcium—The most abundant mineral in the body, which is essential for constriction of blood vessels, normal heart beat, nerve impulses, blood clotting, and many chemical reactions.

Calcium-channel blocker—A drug that blocks the entry of calcium into the smooth muscles of arteries and arterioles, thereby preventing their constriction and causing them to dilate and lower blood pressure. Some of these drugs also depress the rate and contractility of the heart.

Capillaries—Minute vessels connecting arterioles and venules, forming networks throughout the body tissues, which permit exchange of substances between the blood and tissue fluid.

Cardiovascular—Involving the heart (cardio) and blood vessels (vascular).

Carotene—A substance found in many plants (especially carrots) that is changed into vitamin A.

Carotenoids—A group of substances with red or yellow pigment, contained in animal fat and some plants.

CAT (or CT) scan—Computerized axial tomography, an X-ray technique that records many images of the body in multiple planes (views).

Cessation—Discontinuance.

Cholesterol—A fat-like substance (lipid) used especially to build cell membranes and make some hormones. It is present only in animal tissues and dairy products (such as eggs, milk, and butter). Cholesterol is made in the liver and absorbed from food in the intestine. It is transported in the blood mainly as LDL (low-density lipoprotein—the "bad" cholesterol) and HDL (high-density lipoprotein—the "good" cholesterol).

Claudication—Pain or fatigue of muscles, particularly that experienced in the leg muscles on walking, caused by inadequate circulation usually resulting from atherosclerosis of the arteries supplying the muscles. Sometimes referred to as "intermittent claudication," because it is induced by walking and relieved by rest.

Coarctation—A congenital, localized constriction or narrowing of the aorta resulting in hypertension in the upper body (above the constriction) and low blood pressure in the lower body (below the constriction).

Congestive heart failure—Results from diseases or conditions (hypertension, coronary disease, myocardial infarction, valvular disease, inflammation, and so on) that impair the pumping efficiency of the heart and causes accumulation of blood and fluid in the lungs and usually elsewhere in the body.

Constriction—A narrowing of the caliber—for example, in arteries and arterioles due to contraction of smooth muscle cells. This constriction elevates blood pressure.

Contraindication—Any condition that makes a treatment undesirable and inadvisable.

Coronary artery disease—Damage of the arteries supplying blood to the heart muscle, usually the result of cholesterol plaques on the lining of the arteries, which impairs blood supply and may cause angina (chest pressure or pain) or heart attack.

Cushing's syndrome—A condition resulting from excessive amounts of an adrenal hormone (cortisol) in the blood or from excess administration of a synthetic hormone (corticosteroid), which results in an altered body appearance and often hypertension.

DASH—An acronym for Dietary Approach to Stop Hypertension.

Diabetes mellitus—A condition causing elevation of blood sugar due to lack of insulin (type I, occurs in childhood) or resistance to the effect of insulin metabolism (type II, adult onset diabetes).

Dialysis (hemodialysis)—A method of removing elevated levels of waste products and undesirable chemicals from the blood of patients with severe kidney failure. Blood can be continuously passed through an artificial kidney containing dialyzing fluid, or dialyzing fluid can be continuously introduced into and removed from the peritoneal cavity (abdomen) to "cleanse" the blood and restore it to a more normal composition.

Diastole—The period between beats when the heart is at rest and not contracting.

Diastolic blood pressure—The pressure between beats, when the heart is not contracting; it is the lower of the two numbers recorded as the blood pressure.

Diuretic—A drug that causes the kidney to excrete increased amounts of salt and water and lowers blood pressure.

DNA—Deoxyribonucleic acid. This class of nucleic acids, which are found chiefly in the nucleus of cells, causes transference of genetic characteristics and synthesis of proteins.

Doppler ultrasonography—A technique using ultrasound waves to determine blood flow.

Echocardiogram—A diagnostic technique using an instrument that is moved about on the chest and employs sonar (echo) waves to visualize abnormalities in the anatomy or the function of the heart and its valves.

Eclampsia—A serious condition occurring in late pregnancy, which follows preeclampsia, with marked elevation of blood pressure, retention of fluid, sometimes convulsive seizures, and occasionally death of the mother and fetus.

Elaborate—To produce.

Elastic recoil of the aorta—The return to the normal caliber of the aorta after being distended by blood pumped into it from the heart. The return to normal caliber depends on the "elastic" quality of the aorta.

Electrocardiogram (ECG or EKG)—A graphic display of the electrical activity of the heart, recorded from electrodes on the chest and extremities.

Embolus—A clot, brought by the blood from another location where it originated, that obstructs the circulation.

Enzyme—A protein that speeds up a chemical reaction.

ESRD—End-stage renal disease; very severe kidney failure.

Essential hypertension—Also called primary hypertension, it accounts for almost 95% of the hypertensive population. The cause of essential hypertension remains unknown.

Fecal—Pertaining to the excrement discharged from the intestine (feces).

Fetus—The developing young in the uterus after the second month of pregnancy.

Fibromuscular dysplasia—A constriction or constrictions of an artery supplying the kidney that can lead to impaired blood supply to the kidney, with subsequent release of renin and development of hypertension.

Free radical—A damaging chemical, usually an oxidation by-product, that is thought to damage the lining of arteries and possibly play a role in causing cancer.

Generic drug—A drug that is not protected by a patent. Its name is usually descriptive of its chemical composition, and the drug is typically less expensive than its brand-name counterpart but equally effective in causing a response.

Homocysteine—An amino acid (a substance used by the body to make proteins) that, when elevated in the blood, is believed to cause damage and hardening of the arteries (atherosclerosis).

Hormone—A substance released from a gland (such as the adrenal or thyroid gland) or cells in one part of the body, which is transported in the blood and affects distant organs or cells. Examples include adrenaline, noradrenaline, and thyroxin.

Hyperaldosteronism—An increase in the level of aldosterone, a hormone that is secreted from the adrenal gland and causes retention of sodium and water by the kidney; overproduction of aldosterone produces hypertension.

Hyperlability—Marked instability; high changeability.

Hyperthyroidism—Overactivity of the thyroid gland with increased secretion of thyroid hormones, which can cause many signs and symptoms, including hypertension (usually systolic).

Hypertrophy—An enlargement or overgrowth of an organ or tissue.

Hypotension—Abnormally low blood pressure that can cause light-headedness, weakness, blurred vision, fainting, and unconsciousness.

Hypothyroidism—A decreased activity of the thyroid gland accompanied by deficient release of thyroid hormone, which results in a variety of manifestations and sometimes hypertension.

Imaging—The production of images by radiologic, ultrasound, or magnetic resonance imaging (MRI) techniques.

Imaging techniques—Techniques (such as CAT scan, MRI, X rays, ultrasound, and radioactive scans) that permit visualizing (seeing) areas of the body.

Impedance to blood flow—Resistance to blood flow such as that occurring when vessels become constricted.

Impotence—The inability to develop and/or sustain an erection and perform sexual intercourse.

Intermittent claudication—Pain experienced in the lower extremities and sometimes in the hips and buttocks on walking due to diminished blood supply, usually caused by atherosclerosis.

Ischemia—An inadequate blood supply to a part of the body.

Labile hypertension—Blood pressure that may be normal sometimes and hypertensive at other times; fluctuations are especially pronounced.

LDL—Low-density lipoprotein cholesterol. Also known as the "bad" cholesterol, because it can deposit cholesterol on the lining of blood vessels and cause obstructive plaques and atherosclerosis.

Left ventricular hypertrophy (LVH)—Enlargement of the muscle of the left (main) pumping chamber of the heart, which can result from hypertension because of the extra work required to pump blood effectively against elevated blood pressure.

Libido—Sexual desire.

Liddle's syndrome—A genetic abnormality of the kidney, which retains sodium and excretes potassium in excessive amounts.

Lipids—A general term for fats that includes the various types of cholesterol and the triglycerides.

Lipoprotein—A combination of a lipid and protein.

Lupus—A chronic disease of unknown cause, which can involve many tissues in the body, including the skin, lungs, kidneys, and joints.

Magnesium—A mineral in the body that is required for many chemical reactions. A deficiency of magnesium causes irritability of the nervous system.

Metabolize—To biochemically build up or utilize substances to permit growth and energy in the body.

mm Hg—Millimeters (mm) of mercury (Hg); a volume of Hg is 13.5 times heavier than the same volume of water. Blood pressure is expressed as mm Hg elevated in a glass tube recorded with a sphygmomanometer.

MRI—Magnetic resonance imaging; an imaging technique employing magnetic energy rather than X rays.

Multi-infarct dementia—A disorder that arises when multiple areas of the brain suffer damage caused by multiple strokes with impairment of brain function (e.g., memory and judgment deterioration, personality changes).

Murmur—A blowing sound, often heard with a stethoscope over various areas of the heart (usually caused by abnormal heart valves) or over narrowed arteries. Sounds vary in quality and loudness and result from a disturbed blood flow.

Myocardial infarction—An area of dead heart muscle caused by impairment of blood supply, usually due to blockage of a coronary artery.

Neurohormone—A hormone used in the function of the nervous system. For example, noradrenaline is the neurohormone mainly responsible for the function of sympathetic nerves.

Nitric oxide (NO)—A substance released from the cells lining arteries and arterioles, which causes relaxation of smooth muscle and dilation of the vessels.

Noradrenaline—A neurohormone released from sympathetic nerve endings and the adrenal gland, which can cause hypertension by constricting arteries and arterioles and can increase the rate and contraction of the heart.

NSAIDs—Nonsteroidal anti-inflammatory drugs. NSAIDs include aspirin and aspirin-like drugs (e.g., Indacin, Motrin, Advil, Clinoril, Naprosyn). They block the enzyme responsible for the body's synthesis of prostaglandins and related substances. Blocking synthesis of some prostaglandins can cause salt and water retention by the kidney and thereby increase blood pressure.

Ophthalmoscope—An instrument used to examine the interior of the eye.

Osteoporosis—An abnormal decrease in bone density—namely, a thinning and loss of calcium and bone substance.

Pallor—Paleness or decrease in skin coloration in Caucasians.

Palpable—Felt by touching.

Papilledema—Swelling of the optic nerve that can be seen in the back of the eye with an ophthalmoscope; it may occur when the blood pressure is severely elevated.

Parathyroid glands—Four small glands situated in the neck beside the thyroid gland. These glands secrete parathyroid hormone, which is mainly concerned with calcium and phosphorus metabolism.

Pheochromocytoma—A rare tumor that most frequently occurs in an adrenal gland but may occur elsewhere; it usually secretes adrenaline and noradrenaline, which cause many manifestations including hypertension.

Pituitary gland—A small gland at the base of the brain that secretes substances that affect hormone production and bodily functions.

Placebo—A "dummy," innocuous medical treatment used as a control when evaluating a drug or procedure. If the drug or procedure is effective, it should produce better results than a placebo.

Platelets—Very small, cell-like structures in the circulation that are involved in blood clotting.

Postural hypotension—An abnormal decrease in blood pressure on standing, which may be associated with lightheadedness, weakness, and fainting.

Preeclampsia—A condition of unknown cause occurring in about 3% of individuals during the last three months of pregnancy, accompanied by hypertension, fluid retention, and proteinuria.

Primary hypertension—See *Essential hypertension.*

Prognosis—A forecast or predicted outcome of a disease; the prospects of recovery.

Prostaglandins— A group of chemicals that are synthesized in the body. Some can cause dilation of arterioles, whereas others can cause constriction and thereby affect blood pressure. Prostaglandins can also influence blood clotting. Their synthesis can be blocked by aspirin and other NSAIDs (nonsteroidal anti-inflammatory drugs).

Pulse pressure—The difference between systolic and diastolic pressure (subtract the diastolic pressure from the systolic pressure).

Receptor—A structure on a cell that can be stimulated by a specific hormone or chemical to cause a biological response.

Renal—Related to the kidney.

Renal artery stenosis—Narrowing of an artery to a kidney that, if severe, may cause hypertension by increasing renin. The renin then generates angiotensin II, a powerful constrictor of arterioles.

Renin—An enzyme that is released from the kidney into the circulation and generates angiotensin I (an inactive substance), which is then converted to angiotensin II, a powerful constrictor of arteries and arterioles that can elevate blood pressure.

Resistant hypertension—Hypertension that does not appear to respond to lifestyle changes and drug treatment.

Risk factors (of hypertension)—Factors that increase the risk of heart, brain, kidney, eye, and vascular damage.

Secrete—Elaborate, give off, or produce.

Sleep apnea—A periodic cessation of air flow through the mouth and nose during sleep.

Sodium—A mineral that makes up 40% of sodium chloride, which is commonly used as table salt, in cooking, and in processed food. Some salt-sensitive persons retain excess salt and water, which can cause hypertension.

Sphygmomanometer—An instrument used for measuring arterial blood pressure.

Stenosis—A narrowing or constriction.

Stethoscope—An instrument used to listen to sounds made by the heart, the lungs, and arterial narrowing or pulsations (including sounds in the arm during blood pressure measurement).

Stimulate—To excite and cause increased activity.

Stress test—A type of test used to evaluate the effect of exercise on the electrical activity and function of the heart and on the blood flow in the coronary arteries.

Stroke—Sudden brain injury due to inadequate blood supply, resulting from a blocked artery or hemorrhage due to a ruptured artery. Brain damage may be large or minimal, following a small temporary blockage such as a TIA (a "ministroke").

Stroke-prone rats—Rats that have a greater tendency to develop stroke than other rats when they become hypertensive.

Sympathetic nervous system—Part of the autonomic or "involuntary" nervous system over which we have no control. It consists of nerves that release noradrenaline, which constricts arteries and arterioles and increases the rate and force of heart contractions, thereby elevating blood pressure.

Systole—Contraction of the heart, which pumps blood into the aorta.

Systolic blood pressure—The pressure during systole, when the heart is contracting to pump blood into the aorta. It is the higher of the two numbers used to record blood pressure.

Target organs—Organs that can be damaged by hypertension, especially arteries of the heart, brain, kidney, eye, and lower extremities.

Therapeutic—Having a beneficial or curative effect.

Therapy—Treatment.

Thromboxane—A substance in the body that causes constriction of blood vessels and aggregation (clumping) of platelets.

Thyroid gland—A gland occurring in the front of the neck that secretes thyroid hormones, which are important in body metabolism.

Transient ischemic attack (TIA)—A temporary inadequate blood supply to an area of the brain, which causes transient neurological manifestations, often due to a "ministroke" caused by a small blood clot.

Triglycerides—Lipids (fats) in the blood that, if elevated, may contribute to atherosclerosis; severe elevations may also cause pancreatitis, an inflammation of the pancreas.

TSH—Thyroid-stimulating hormone; a hormone released from the pituitary gland that stimulates thyroid function.

Uremia—Excess accumulation of waste products and chemicals in the blood because of kidney failure and the inability to adequately excrete these substances in the urine.

Vascular—Related to the vascular system, which is composed of blood vessels made up of large and small arteries, which are in turn connected by capillaries to small and large veins.

Vasoconstrictor—A substance that constricts (i.e., narrows) blood vessels; constriction can be caused by substances normally present in the body and by some medications. Vasoconstriction of arterioles is mainly responsible for elevating blood pressure.

Vasodilator—A substance that causes dilation (i.e., expansion) of blood vessels; dilation can be caused by substances normally present in the body and by some medications. Vasodilation of arterioles is mainly responsible for lowering blood pressure.

Vasopeptidase inhibitor—A member of a new class of antihypertensive drugs that are particularly effective in lowering systolic blood pressure. Vasopeptidase inhibitors offer dual effects: they act as ACE inhibitors, and they block the degradation of certain hormones that dilate blood vessels and that eliminate salt and water.

Veins—Blood vessels that return blood from the body and the lungs to the heart. Blood returning from the body requires replenishing of its oxygen content, which was removed by the tissues. Blood is oxygenated in the lungs and then returned to the left ventricle, which pumps it into the aorta.

Ventricle—One of two large pumping chambers of the heart. The right ventricle pumps blood to the lungs, whereas the left ventricle, which has a muscle wall three times thicker than that of the right ventricle, pumps blood to all parts of the body.

Vitamin—A general term for substances that occur in many plant and animal foods and that are necessary in extremely small amounts for normal body function.

White-coat hypertension—Hypertension that occurs in the doctor's office but does not occur at home or elsewhere. Anxiety and fear in the doctor's office are probably responsible for this type of transient hypertension.

Index

Note: Page numbers followed by *f* refer to illustrations; page numbers followed by *t* refer to tables.